Mometrix
TEST PREPARATION

Renal Nutrition Exam Secrets Study Guide

AF901458

DEAR FUTURE EXAM SUCCESS STORY

First of all, **THANK YOU** for purchasing Mometrix study materials!

Second, congratulations! You are one of the few determined test-takers who are committed to doing whatever it takes to excel on your exam. **You have come to the right place.** We developed these study materials with one goal in mind: to deliver you the information you need in a format that's concise and easy to use.

In addition to optimizing your guide for the content of the test, we've outlined our recommended steps for breaking down the preparation process into small, attainable goals so you can make sure you stay on track.

We've also analyzed the entire test-taking process, identifying the most common pitfalls and showing how you can overcome them and be ready for any curveball the test throws you.

Standardized testing is one of the biggest obstacles on your road to success, which only increases the importance of doing well in the high-pressure, high-stakes environment of test day. Your results on this test could have a significant impact on your future, and this guide provides the information and practical advice to help you achieve your full potential on test day.

Your success is our success

We would love to hear from you! If you would like to share the story of your exam success or if you have any questions or comments in regard to our products, please contact us at **800-673-8175** or **support@mometrix.com**.

Thanks again for your business and we wish you continued success!

Sincerely,
The Mometrix Test Preparation Team

Need more help? Check out our flashcards at:
http://MometrixFlashcards.com/Nutrition

Written and edited by the Mometrix Exam Secrets Test Prep Team
Printed in the United States of America

Table of Contents

Introduction

Thank you for purchasing this resource! You have made the choice to prepare yourself for a test that could have a huge impact on your future, and this guide is designed to help you be fully ready for test day. Obviously, it's important to have a solid understanding of the test material, but you also need to be prepared for the unique environment and stressors of the test, so that you can perform to the best of your abilities.

For this purpose, the first section that appears in this guide is the **Secret Keys**. We've devoted countless hours to meticulously researching what works and what doesn't, and we've boiled down our findings to the five most impactful steps you can take to improve your performance on the test. We start at the beginning with study planning and move through the preparation process, all the way to the testing strategies that will help you get the most out of what you know when you're finally sitting in front of the test.

We recommend that you start preparing for your test as far in advance as possible. However, if you've bought this guide as a last-minute study resource and only have a few days before your test, we recommend that you skip over the first two Secret Keys since they address a long-term study plan.

If you struggle with **test anxiety**, we strongly encourage you to check out our recommendations for how you can overcome it. Test anxiety is a formidable foe, but it can be beaten, and we want to make sure you have the tools you need to defeat it.

Secret Key 1: Plan Big, Study Small

There's a lot riding on your performance. If you want to ace this test, you're going to need to keep your skills sharp and the material fresh in your mind. You need a plan that lets you review everything you need to know while still fitting in your schedule. We'll break this strategy down into three categories.

Information Organization

Start with the information you already have: the official test outline. From this, you can make a complete list of all the concepts you need to cover before the test. Organize these concepts into groups that can be studied together, and create a list of any related vocabulary you need to learn so you can brush up on any difficult terms. You'll want to keep this vocabulary list handy once you actually start studying since you may need to add to it along the way.

Time Management

Once you have your set of study concepts, decide how to spread them out over the time you have left before the test. Break your study plan into small, clear goals so you have a manageable task for each day and know exactly what you're doing. Then just focus on one small step at a time. When you manage your time this way, you don't need to spend hours at a time studying. Studying a small block of content for a short period each day helps you retain information better and avoid stressing over how much you have left to do. You can relax knowing that you have a plan to cover everything in time. In order for this strategy to be effective though, you have to start studying early and stick to your schedule. Avoid the exhaustion and futility that comes from last-minute cramming!

Study Environment

The environment you study in has a big impact on your learning. Studying in a coffee shop, while probably more enjoyable, is not likely to be as fruitful as studying in a quiet room. It's important to keep distractions to a minimum. You're only planning to study for a short block of time, so make the most of it. Don't pause to check your phone or get up to find a snack. It's also important to **avoid multitasking**. Research has consistently shown that multitasking will make your studying dramatically less effective. Your study area should also be comfortable and well-lit so you don't have the distraction of straining your eyes or sitting on an uncomfortable chair.

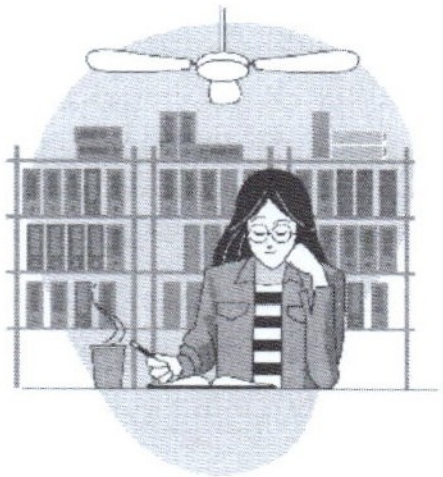

The time of day you study is also important. You want to be rested and alert. Don't wait until just before bedtime. Study when you'll be most likely to comprehend and remember. Even better, if you know what time of day your test will be, set that time aside for study. That way your brain will be used to working on that subject at that specific time and you'll have a better chance of recalling information.

Finally, it can be helpful to team up with others who are studying for the same test. Your actual studying should be done in as isolated an environment as possible, but the work of organizing the information and setting up the study plan can be divided up. In between study sessions, you can discuss with your teammates the concepts that you're all studying and quiz each other on the details. Just be sure that your teammates are as serious about the test as you are. If you find that your study time is being replaced with social time, you might need to find a new team.

Secret Key 2: Make Your Studying Count

You're devoting a lot of time and effort to preparing for this test, so you want to be absolutely certain it will pay off. This means doing more than just reading the content and hoping you can remember it on test day. It's important to make every minute of study count. There are two main areas you can focus on to make your studying count.

Retention

It doesn't matter how much time you study if you can't remember the material. You need to make sure you are retaining the concepts. To check your retention of the information you're learning, try recalling it at later times with minimal prompting. Try carrying around flashcards and glance at one or two from time to time or ask a friend who's also studying for the test to quiz you.

To enhance your retention, look for ways to put the information into practice so that you can apply it rather than simply recalling it. If you're using the information in practical ways, it will be much easier to remember. Similarly, it helps to solidify a concept in your mind if you're not only reading it to yourself but also explaining it to someone else. Ask a friend to let you teach them about a concept you're a little shaky on (or speak aloud to an imaginary audience if necessary). As you try to summarize, define, give examples, and answer your friend's questions, you'll understand the concepts better and they will stay with you longer. Finally, step back for a big picture view and ask yourself how each piece of information fits with the whole subject. When you link the different concepts together and see them working together as a whole, it's easier to remember the individual components.

Finally, practice showing your work on any multi-step problems, even if you're just studying. Writing out each step you take to solve a problem will help solidify the process in your mind, and you'll be more likely to remember it during the test.

Modality

Modality simply refers to the means or method by which you study. Choosing a study modality that fits your own individual learning style is crucial. No two people learn best in exactly the same way, so it's important to know your strengths and use them to your advantage.

For example, if you learn best by visualization, focus on visualizing a concept in your mind and draw an image or a diagram. Try color-coding your notes, illustrating them, or creating symbols that will trigger your mind to recall a learned concept. If you learn best by hearing or discussing information, find a study partner who learns the same way or read aloud to yourself. Think about how to put the information in your own words. Imagine that you are giving a lecture on the topic and record yourself so you can listen to it later.

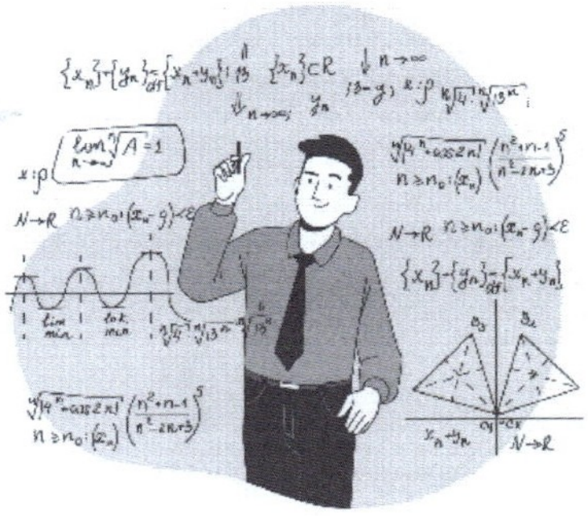

For any learning style, flashcards can be helpful. Organize the information so you can take advantage of spare moments to review. Underline key words or phrases. Use different colors for different categories. Mnemonic devices (such as creating a short list in which every item starts with the same letter) can also help with retention. Find what works best for you and use it to store the information in your mind most effectively and easily.

Secret Key 3: Practice the Right Way

Your success on test day depends not only on how many hours you put into preparing, but also on whether you prepared the right way. It's good to check along the way to see if your studying is paying off. One of the most effective ways to do this is by taking practice tests to evaluate your progress. Practice tests are useful because they show exactly where you need to improve. Every time you take a practice test, pay special attention to these three groups of questions:

- The questions you got wrong
- The questions you had to guess on, even if you guessed right
- The questions you found difficult or slow to work through

This will show you exactly what your weak areas are, and where you need to devote more study time. Ask yourself why each of these questions gave you trouble. Was it because you didn't understand the material? Was it because you didn't remember the vocabulary? Do you need more repetitions on this type of question to build speed and confidence? Dig into those questions and figure out how you can strengthen your weak areas as you go back to review the material.

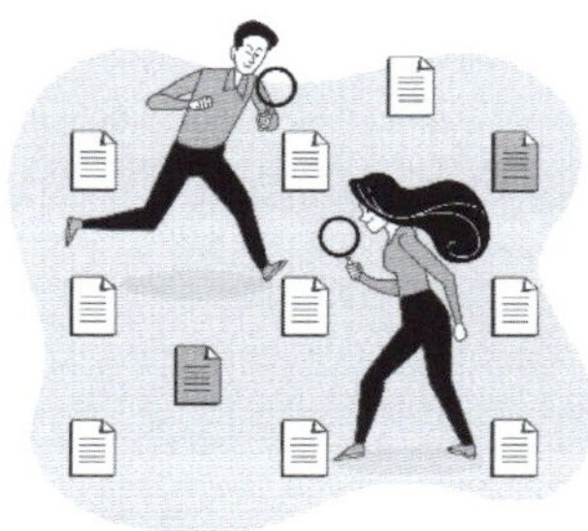

Additionally, many practice tests have a section explaining the answer choices. It can be tempting to read the explanation and think that you now have a good understanding of the concept. However, an explanation likely only covers part of the question's broader context. Even if the explanation makes perfect sense, **go back and investigate** every concept related to the question until you're positive you have a thorough understanding.

As you go along, keep in mind that the practice test is just that: practice. Memorizing these questions and answers will not be very helpful on the actual test because it is unlikely to have any of the same exact questions. If you only know the right answers to the sample questions, you won't be prepared for the real thing. **Study the concepts** until you understand them fully, and then you'll be able to answer any question that shows up on the test.

It's important to wait on the practice tests until you're ready. If you take a test on your first day of study, you may be overwhelmed by the amount of material covered and how much you need to learn. Work up to it gradually.

On test day, you'll need to be prepared for answering questions, managing your time, and using the test-taking strategies you've learned. It's a lot to balance, like a mental marathon that will have a big impact on your future. Like training for a marathon, you'll need to start slowly and work your way up. When test day arrives, you'll be ready.

Start with the strategies you've read in the first two Secret Keys—plan your course and study in the way that works best for you. If you have time, consider using multiple study resources to get different approaches to the same concepts. It can be helpful to see difficult concepts from more than one angle. Then find a good source for practice tests. Many times, the test website will suggest potential study resources or provide sample tests.

Practice Test Strategy

If you're able to find at least three practice tests, we recommend this strategy:

Untimed and Open-Book Practice

Take the first test with no time constraints and with your notes and study guide handy. Take your time and focus on applying the strategies you've learned.

Timed and Open-Book Practice

Take the second practice test open-book as well, but set a timer and practice pacing yourself to finish in time.

Timed and Closed-Book Practice

Take any other practice tests as if it were test day. Set a timer and put away your study materials. Sit at a table or desk in a quiet room, imagine yourself at the testing center, and answer questions as quickly and accurately as possible.

Keep repeating timed and closed-book tests on a regular basis until you run out of practice tests or it's time for the actual test. Your mind will be ready for the schedule and stress of test day, and you'll be able to focus on recalling the material you've learned.

Secret Key 4: Pace Yourself

Once you're fully prepared for the material on the test, your biggest challenge on test day will be managing your time. Just knowing that the clock is ticking can make you panic even if you have plenty of time left. Work on pacing yourself so you can build confidence against the time constraints of the exam. Pacing is a difficult skill to master, especially in a high-pressure environment, so **practice is vital**.

Set time expectations for your pace based on how much time is available. For example, if a section has 60 questions and the time limit is 30 minutes, you know you have to average 30 seconds or less per question in order to answer them all. Although 30 seconds is the hard limit, set 25 seconds per question as your goal, so you reserve extra time to spend on harder questions. When you budget extra time for the harder questions, you no longer have any reason to stress when those questions take longer to answer.

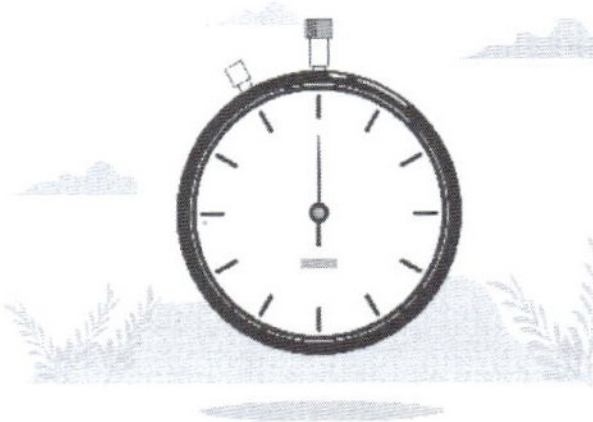

Don't let this time expectation distract you from working through the test at a calm, steady pace, but keep it in mind so you don't spend too much time on any one question. Recognize that taking extra time on one question you don't understand may keep you from answering two that you do understand later in the test. If your time limit for a question is up and you're still not sure of the answer, mark it and move on, and come back to it later if the time and the test format allow. If the testing format doesn't allow you to return to earlier questions, just make an educated guess; then put it out of your mind and move on.

On the easier questions, be careful not to rush. It may seem wise to hurry through them so you have more time for the challenging ones, but it's not worth missing one if you know the concept and just didn't take the time to read the question fully. Work efficiently but make sure you understand the question and have looked at all of the answer choices, since more than one may seem right at first.

Even if you're paying attention to the time, you may find yourself a little behind at some point. You should speed up to get back on track, but do so wisely. Don't panic; just take a few seconds less on each question until you're caught up. Don't guess without thinking, but do look through the answer choices and eliminate any you know are wrong. If you can get down to two choices, it is often worthwhile to guess from those. Once you've chosen an answer, move on and don't dwell on any that you skipped or had to hurry through. If a question was taking too long, chances are it was one of the harder ones, so you weren't as likely to get it right anyway.

On the other hand, if you find yourself getting ahead of schedule, it may be beneficial to slow down a little. The more quickly you work, the more likely you are to make a careless mistake that will affect your score. You've budgeted time for each question, so don't be afraid to spend that time. Practice an efficient but careful pace to get the most out of the time you have.

Secret Key 5: Have a Plan for Guessing

When you're taking the test, you may find yourself stuck on a question. Some of the answer choices seem better than others, but you don't see the one answer choice that is obviously correct. What do you do?

The scenario described above is very common, yet most test takers have not effectively prepared for it. Developing and practicing a plan for guessing may be one of the single most effective uses of your time as you get ready for the exam.

In developing your plan for guessing, there are three questions to address:

- When should you start the guessing process?
- How should you narrow down the choices?
- Which answer should you choose?

When to Start the Guessing Process

Unless your plan for guessing is to select C every time (which, despite its merits, is not what we recommend), you need to leave yourself enough time to apply your answer elimination strategies. Since you have a limited amount of time for each question, that means that if you're going to give yourself the best shot at guessing correctly, you have to decide quickly whether or not you will guess.

Of course, the best-case scenario is that you don't have to guess at all, so first, see if you can answer the question based on your knowledge of the subject and basic reasoning skills. Focus on the key words in the question and try to jog your memory of related topics. Give yourself a chance to bring the knowledge to mind, but once you realize that you don't have (or you can't access) the knowledge you need to answer the question, it's time to start the guessing process.

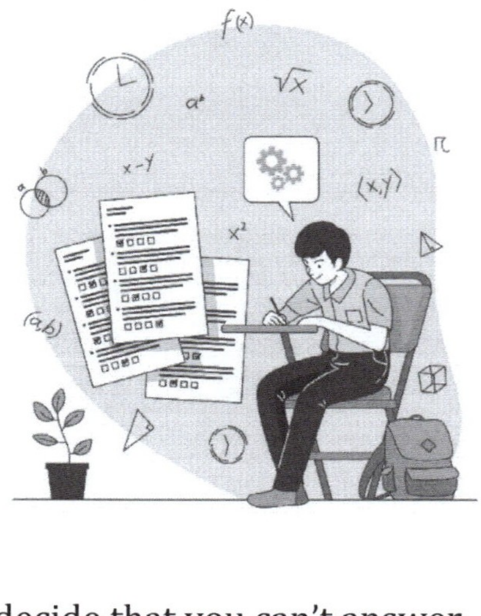

It's almost always better to start the guessing process too early than too late. It only takes a few seconds to remember something and answer the question from knowledge. Carefully eliminating wrong answer choices takes longer. Plus, going through the process of eliminating answer choices can actually help jog your memory.

Summary: Start the guessing process as soon as you decide that you can't answer the question based on your knowledge.

How to Narrow Down the Choices

The next chapter in this book (**Test-Taking Strategies**) includes a wide range of strategies for how to approach questions and how to look for answer choices to eliminate. You will definitely want to read those carefully, practice them, and figure out which ones work best for you. Here though, we're going to address a mindset rather than a particular strategy.

Your odds of guessing an answer correctly depend on how many options you are choosing from.

Number of options left	5	4	3	2	1
Odds of guessing correctly	20%	25%	33%	50%	100%

You can see from this chart just how valuable it is to be able to eliminate incorrect answers and make an educated guess, but there are two things that many test takers do that cause them to miss out on the benefits of guessing:

- Accidentally eliminating the correct answer
- Selecting an answer based on an impression

We'll look at the first one here, and the second one in the next section.

To avoid accidentally eliminating the correct answer, we recommend a thought exercise called **the $5 challenge**. In this challenge, you only eliminate an answer choice from contention if you are willing to bet $5 on it being wrong. Why $5? Five dollars is a small but not insignificant amount of money. It's an amount you could afford to lose but wouldn't want to throw away. And while losing $5 once might not hurt too much, doing it twenty times will set you back $100. In the same way, each small decision you make—eliminating a choice here, guessing on a question there—won't by itself impact your score very much, but when you put them all together, they can make a big difference. By holding each answer choice elimination decision to a higher standard, you can reduce the risk of accidentally eliminating the correct answer.

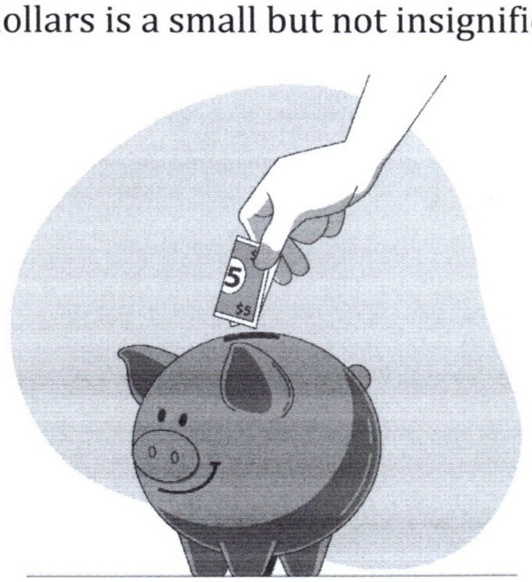

The $5 challenge can also be applied in a positive sense: If you are willing to bet $5 that an answer choice *is* correct, go ahead and mark it as correct.

Summary: Only eliminate an answer choice if you are willing to bet $5 that it is wrong.

Which Answer to Choose

You're taking the test. You've run into a hard question and decided you'll have to guess. You've eliminated all the answer choices you're willing to bet $5 on. Now you have to pick an answer. Why do we even need to talk about this? Why can't you just pick whichever one you feel like when the time comes?

The answer to these questions is that if you don't come into the test with a plan, you'll rely on your impression to select an answer choice, and if you do that, you risk falling into a trap. The test writers know that everyone who takes their test will be guessing on some of the questions, so they intentionally write wrong answer choices to seem plausible. You still have to pick an answer though, and if the wrong answer choices are designed to look right, how can you ever be sure that you're not falling for their trap? The best solution we've found to this dilemma is to take the decision out of your hands entirely. Here is the process we recommend:

Once you've eliminated any choices that you are confident (willing to bet $5) are wrong, select the first remaining choice as your answer.

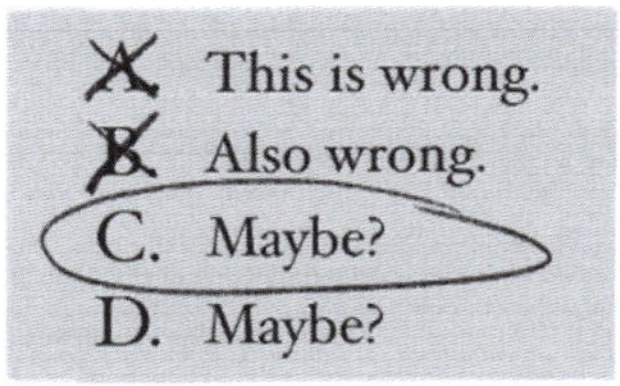

Whether you choose to select the first remaining choice, the second, or the last, the important thing is that you use some preselected standard. Using this approach guarantees that you will not be enticed into selecting an answer choice that looks right, because you are not basing your decision on how the answer choices look.

This is not meant to make you question your knowledge. Instead, it is to help you recognize the difference between your knowledge and your impressions. There's a huge difference between thinking an answer is right because of what you know, and thinking an answer is right because it looks or sounds like it should be right.

Summary: To ensure that your selection is appropriately random, make a predetermined selection from among all answer choices you have not eliminated.

Test-Taking Strategies

This section contains a list of test-taking strategies that you may find helpful as you work through the test. By taking what you know and applying logical thought, you can maximize your chances of answering any question correctly!

It is very important to realize that every question is different and every person is different: no single strategy will work on every question, and no single strategy will work for every person. That's why we've included all of them here, so you can try them out and determine which ones work best for different types of questions and which ones work best for you.

Question Strategies

☑ Read Carefully

Read the question and the answer choices carefully. Don't miss the question because you misread the terms. You have plenty of time to read each question thoroughly and make sure you understand what is being asked. Yet a happy medium must be attained, so don't waste too much time. You must read carefully and efficiently.

☑ Contextual Clues

Look for contextual clues. If the question includes a word you are not familiar with, look at the immediate context for some indication of what the word might mean. Contextual clues can often give you all the information you need to decipher the meaning of an unfamiliar word. Even if you can't determine the meaning, you may be able to narrow down the possibilities enough to make a solid guess at the answer to the question.

☑ Prefixes

If you're having trouble with a word in the question or answer choices, try dissecting it. Take advantage of every clue that the word might include. Prefixes can be a huge help. Usually, they allow you to determine a basic meaning. *Pre-* means before, *post-* means after, *pro-* is positive, *de-* is negative. From prefixes, you can get an idea of the general meaning of the word and try to put it into context.

☑ Hedge Words

Watch out for critical hedge words, such as *likely, may, can, often, almost, mostly, usually, generally, rarely,* and *sometimes.* Question writers insert these hedge phrases to cover every possibility. Often an answer choice will be wrong simply because it leaves no room for exception. Be on guard for answer choices that have definitive words such as *exactly* and *always.*

☑ Switchback Words

Stay alert for *switchbacks*. These are the words and phrases frequently used to alert you to shifts in thought. The most common switchback words are *but*, *although*, and *however*. Others include *nevertheless, on the other hand, even though, while, in spite of, despite*, and *regardless of*. Switchback words are important to catch because they can change the direction of the question or an answer choice.

☑ Face Value

When in doubt, use common sense. Accept the situation in the problem at face value. Don't read too much into it. These problems will not require you to make wild assumptions. If you have to go beyond creativity and warp time or space in order to have an answer choice fit the question, then you should move on and consider the other answer choices. These are normal problems rooted in reality. The applicable relationship or explanation may not be readily apparent, but it is there for you to figure out. Use your common sense to interpret anything that isn't clear.

Answer Choice Strategies

☑ Answer Selection

The most thorough way to pick an answer choice is to identify and eliminate wrong answers until only one is left, then confirm it is the correct answer. Sometimes an answer choice may immediately seem right, but be careful. The test writers will usually put more than one reasonable answer choice on each question, so take a second to read all of them and make sure that the other choices are not equally obvious. As long as you have time left, it is better to read every answer choice than to pick the first one that looks right without checking the others.

☑ Answer Choice Families

An answer choice family consists of two (in rare cases, three) answer choices that are very similar in construction and cannot all be true at the same time. If you see two answer choices that are direct opposites or parallels, one of them is usually the correct answer. For instance, if one answer choice says that quantity x increases and another either says that quantity x decreases (opposite) or says that quantity y increases (parallel), then those answer choices would fall into the same family. An answer choice that doesn't match the construction of the answer choice family is more likely to be incorrect. Most questions will not have answer choice families, but when they do appear, you should be prepared to recognize them.

☑ Eliminate Answers

Eliminate answer choices as soon as you realize they are wrong, but make sure you consider all possibilities. If you are eliminating answer choices and realize that the last one you are left with is also wrong, don't panic. Start over and consider each choice again. There may be something you missed the first time that you will realize on the second pass.

☑ Avoid Fact Traps

Don't be distracted by an answer choice that is factually true but doesn't answer the question. You are looking for the choice that answers the question. Stay focused on what the question is asking for so you don't accidentally pick an answer that is true but incorrect. Always go back to the question and make sure the answer choice you've selected actually answers the question and is not merely a true statement.

☑ Extreme Statements

In general, you should avoid answers that put forth extreme actions as standard practice or proclaim controversial ideas as established fact. An answer choice that states the "process should be used in certain situations, if..." is much more likely to be correct than one that states the "process should be discontinued completely." The first is a calm rational statement and doesn't even make a definitive, uncompromising stance, using a hedge word *if* to provide wiggle room, whereas the second choice is far more extreme.

☑ Benchmark

As you read through the answer choices and you come across one that seems to answer the question well, mentally select that answer choice. This is not your final answer, but it's the one that will help you evaluate the other answer choices. The one that you selected is your benchmark or standard for judging each of the other answer choices. Every other answer choice must be compared to your benchmark. That choice is correct until proven otherwise by another answer choice beating it. If you find a better answer, then that one becomes your new benchmark. Once you've decided that no other choice answers the question as well as your benchmark, you have your final answer.

☑ Predict the Answer

Before you even start looking at the answer choices, it is often best to try to predict the answer. When you come up with the answer on your own, it is easier to avoid distractions and traps because you will know exactly what to look for. The right answer choice is unlikely to be word-for-word what you came up with, but it should be a close match. Even if you are confident that you have the right answer, you should still take the time to read each option before moving on.

General Strategies

☑ Tough Questions

If you are stumped on a problem or it appears too hard or too difficult, don't waste time. Move on! Remember though, if you can quickly check for obviously incorrect answer choices, your chances of guessing correctly are greatly improved. Before you completely give up, at least try to knock out a couple of possible answers. Eliminate what you can and then guess at the remaining answer choices before moving on.

⊘ Check Your Work

Since you will probably not know every term listed and the answer to every question, it is important that you get credit for the ones that you do know. Don't miss any questions through careless mistakes. If at all possible, try to take a second to look back over your answer selection and make sure you've selected the correct answer choice and haven't made a costly careless mistake (such as marking an answer choice that you didn't mean to mark). This quick double check should more than pay for itself in caught mistakes for the time it costs.

⊘ Pace Yourself

It's easy to be overwhelmed when you're looking at a page full of questions; your mind is confused and full of random thoughts, and the clock is ticking down faster than you would like. Calm down and maintain the pace that you have set for yourself. Especially as you get down to the last few minutes of the test, don't let the small numbers on the clock make you panic. As long as you are on track by monitoring your pace, you are guaranteed to have time for each question.

⊘ Don't Rush

It is very easy to make errors when you are in a hurry. Maintaining a fast pace in answering questions is pointless if it makes you miss questions that you would have gotten right otherwise. Test writers like to include distracting information and wrong answers that seem right. Taking a little extra time to avoid careless mistakes can make all the difference in your test score. Find a pace that allows you to be confident in the answers that you select.

⊘ Keep Moving

Panicking will not help you pass the test, so do your best to stay calm and keep moving. Taking deep breaths and going through the answer elimination steps you practiced can help to break through a stress barrier and keep your pace.

Final Notes

The combination of a solid foundation of content knowledge and the confidence that comes from practicing your plan for applying that knowledge is the key to maximizing your performance on test day. As your foundation of content knowledge is built up and strengthened, you'll find that the strategies included in this chapter become more and more effective in helping you quickly sift through the distractions and traps of the test to isolate the correct answer.

Now that you're preparing to move forward into the test content chapters of this book, be sure to keep your goal in mind. As you read, think about how you will be able to apply this information on the test. If you've already seen sample questions for the test and you have an idea of the question format and style, try to come up with questions of your own that you can answer based on what you're reading. This will give you valuable practice applying your knowledge in the same ways you can expect to on test day.

Good luck and good studying!

Integration of Medical Information

Medical History

Obtaining information about an individual's medical history is an important component of nutrition assessment. Information about current medical conditions affecting health status as well as past medical history is important. A surgical history for recent and past surgeries is also important. Information detailing any gastrointestinal issues is very useful. A detailed family history should be obtained. A history of drug or alcohol use is required as this can significantly impact health. A weight history including recent weight changes should be obtained. For older patients, it is important to complete a more in-depth functional assessment including mental status changes, changes in vision or hearing, changes in physical abilities, and a review of both over-the-counter and prescription drug use.

Risk Factors CKD

There are many different risk factors for developing chronic kidney disease (CKD). Diabetes is a significant risk factor for CKD and may be the cause in approximately 33% of new cases. Hypertension is a second significant risk factor, because the presence of hypertension puts added stress on blood vessels, especially those in the kidney. Another risk factor for CKD is blockage of the genitourinary tract. These can be due to atherosclerosis, blood clots, or scar tissue that forms and causes urine to back up into the kidney causing damage. The excessive use of certain pain medications such as ibuprofen, naproxen, and acetaminophen has been associated with interstitial nephritis that can lead to CKD. Allergic reactions to certain antibiotics such as penicillin or vancomycin can also cause nephritis and lead to CKD. Other types of illegal drugs such as heroin or cocaine can cause major kidney damage over time. Family history and age are also risk factors.

Five Stages of CKD

CKD is classified into one of five stages and is based initially on glomerular filtration rate (GFR) with normal value considered to be above 90 mL/min/1.73 m^2. Additionally, an ultrasound or CT scan of the kidneys will help to determine size or the presence of structural abnormalities. Sometimes a kidney biopsy is needed. The 5 stages are as follows:

- Stage 1- the GFR is greater than 90 but proteinuria is present indicating kidney damage
- Stage 2- a mild reduction in GFR at 60-89
- Stage 3- a moderate reduction in GFR at 30-59
- Stage 4- a severe reduction in GFR at 15-29
- Stage 5- considered to be in kidney failure with dialysis or kidney transplant required; GFR is less than 15

Possible Treatment Plan for a Patient with Stage 5 CKD

Initial treatment for this scenario should be aimed at reducing LDL levels to less than 100 mg/dL. This is important because individuals with CKD have at least a 20% chance of developing coronary heart disease over a 10-year period, which puts this scenario in the highest risk category. Initial treatment involves implementing the Therapeutic Lifestyle Changes (TLC) diet. This is best achieved with the assistance of a registered dietitian (RD). A plan for weight management is essential, and increased physical activity of moderate intensity for at least 20-30 minutes 3 to 4 times per week should be incorporated. Limiting alcohol intake to no more than 1 drink per day with the approval of the patient's physician is recommended. Counseling to stop smoking is especially important. If success is not seen at the 3-month reassessment, treatment with a statin such as lovastatin is advised. Pravastatin or simvastatin is recommended. TLC should continue.

Risk Factors for CVD in Patients with CKD

Cardiovascular disease (CVD) is frequently seen in individuals with CKD. Because of this, there is an increased risk of mortality in this population. Traditional risk factors for CVD in patients with CKD are very similar to those of the general population. Certain risk factors are modifiable while others are not. Risk factors include:

- Hypertension
- Diabetes
- Smoking
- Elevated serum cholesterol, elevated triglycerides, elevated LDL cholesterol
- Left ventricular hypertrophy, can lead to dilated cardiomyopathy and heart failure
- Positive family history for heart disease
- Age
- Lack of physical activity
- Male gender
- Menopausal women

Risk Factors for CVD

There are a number of factors that increase the risk for CVD in individuals with CKD.

- Sleep abnormalities - may be related in part to hypoxemia at night
- Elevated homocysteine levels - this is an independent risk factor in the general population but for patients receiving dialysis, correction of these levels is often difficult
- Oxidative stress - related to inflammation, malnutrition, byproducts of uremia, and to the dialysis process itself.
- Altered metabolism of calcium, phosphorus, vitamin D, and parathyroid hormone - can lead to hypertrophy of the myocardium, increased vascular calcification
- Anemia - may be associated with increased left ventricular hypertrophy

- Malnutrition - associated with inflammation that can increase CVD risk; malnutrition is often present in patients receiving dialysis
- Volume overload - increases cardiac workload

Diabetes

Diabetes occurs when the body no longer produces enough insulin or cannot utilize the insulin it produces. Pre-diabetes is a condition where blood glucose levels are elevated but not at a level high enough to be considered having type 1 or type 2 diabetes. It is often a warning that diabetes will develop within 10 years. A normal fasting blood glucose is 99 mg/dL or lower. A fasting level of 100-125 mg/dL is considered to be pre-diabetes and a level greater than 126 on two occasions is indicative of diabetes. Alternatively, a random blood glucose greater than 200 and symptoms of polyuria, polydipsia, and unplanned weight loss can also indicate diabetes. Patients diagnosed with diabetes should have a hemoglobin A1C level checked at least twice per year with a goal of less than 7%. Up to 30% of individuals with type 1 diabetes and up to 40% of those with type 2 diabetes will develop kidney failure.

Effects of Diabetes on Kidney Function

The effects of diabetes on the kidney take years to manifest, but even individuals with well-controlled blood glucose levels can develop kidney damage. Altered kidney function is typically not seen within the first 10 years after initial diagnosis. Diabetes can damage the small blood vessels in the kidney and will slowly impact kidney function. The first sign of kidney damage is albumin in the urine. Diabetes can also cause nerve damage that may lead to an inability to fully empty the bladder. This in turn can lead to increased pressure or an increase in bacterial infections due to the high sugar content of the urine. Other early symptoms include an increase in nocturnal urination, swelling of the ankles, and high blood pressure. Later symptoms may include headaches, itching, general feeling of malaise, nausea and vomiting, poor appetite, and edema.

Diabetic Nephropathy

Diabetic nephropathy is kidney dysfunction characterized by protein in the urine.

There are a few ways that an individual with diabetes can reduce the risk for developing kidney disease or diabetic nephropathy. This includes tight control of blood glucose, keeping blood pressure well controlled, and monitoring kidney function at least yearly. This would include checking for proteinuria and estimating the glomerular filtration rate (GFR). Two medications are available that may slow the progression of disease, angiotensin-converting enzyme (ACE) inhibitors or angiotensin receptor blocking (ARB) agents. Other ways to help reduce the risk include staying away from nonsteroidal anti-inflammatory drugs (NSAIDs) such as ibuprofen; treating urinary tract infections quickly; keeping well hydrated; and avoiding alcohol. Quitting smoking will also reduce the risk. Minimizing exposure to tests that may damage the kidneys, such as those that use contrast dyes, will also help to reduce the risk. Controlling lipid levels and reducing protein intake may also be advantageous.

Optimal Medical Management for Diabetes and CKD

Optimal medical management includes achieving and maintaining glycemic control. Target levels for HbA1c should be less than 7% to minimize complications. Insulin or oral hypoglycemic agents are typically used. It should be noted that as the glomerular filtration rate (GFR) decreases, the half-life of insulin increases due to reduction in insulin clearance by the kidney. If the insulin regimen is not adjusted, there will be a higher risk for hypoglycemia. Additionally, certain oral sulfonylurea agents will build up in the blood due to kidney failure and will increase the chance for hypoglycemia. Following the appropriate diet prescribed by the physician or registered dietitian (RD) is recommended. Blood pressure should be tightly controlled using medications appropriate for the individual's medical condition coupled with a sodium- restricted diet. Medications may include an antihypertensive and/or a diuretic. Because individuals with diabetic nephropathy typically have elevated lipid levels, following the appropriate diet and using a statin-type medication is often recommended.

General Diet Recommendations for Diabetes Management

Diet recommendations for diabetes management according to the American Diabetes Association are as follows:

- A caloric restriction is advised for individuals with type 2 diabetes to assist in achieving an appropriate body weight.
- Protein should contribute 10%-20% of total calories unless significant nephropathy is present. In this case, limiting protein to 0.8 grams per kg is recommended.
- Fat should contribute no more than 30%-35% of total calories (less than 10% from saturated fat, less than 10% from polyunsaturated fat, and 10%-15% from monounsaturated fat). Cholesterol should be restricted to less than 300 mg per day.
- Carbohydrate should contribute 45%- 60% of total calories and should be mainly in the form of complex carbohydrates. Simple sugars should be avoided as much as possible, and carbohydrate intake should be adjusted accordingly based on blood glucose response. 20-35 grams per day of fiber should be consumed

Alcohol, Tobacco and Recreational Drug

Abuse of alcohol, tobacco, and illegal drugs such as marijuana or cocaine is strongly discouraged in the general healthy population and especially in individuals with chronic kidney disease (CKD). Along with being a risk factor for cardiovascular disease, smoking causes a faster progression of kidney disease. Smoking affects the blood flow to organs such as the kidney and can worsen kidney disease. Smoking is especially bad for people with high blood pressure or diabetes, both of which are risk factors for kidney disease. Alcohol abuse can lead to hypertension and can interfere with medications used for treating hypertension. Although small amounts of alcohol may be beneficial to heart health, heavy drinking may actually increase the risk for heart failure and may lead to damage to other organs such as the liver. Heart failure will indirectly affect kidney function. Illegal drugs can cause hypertension, heart failure, and damage to the kidney.

Hypotension

Hypotension is defined as a drop in blood pressure. A common occurrence in patients receiving hemodialysis, hypotension may occur in up to 30% of patients. Hypotension occurs for a number of reasons, including the following:

- Cardiac reasons, such as diastolic dysfunction as a result of chronic hypertension, or coronary artery disease, or a decrease in heart rate due to changes in filling pressure
- Changes in blood volume as a result of excessive fluid removal during hemodialysis, large intradialytic weight gains, removal of fluid too quickly, the use of a dry target weight that is too low for the individual patient, or using an incorrect dialysis solution, such as one that may be too hypotonic
- Reduced vasoconstriction due to lowered peripheral vascular resistance, improper temperature of the dialysis solution, eating a large meal prior to a hemodialysis session, or anemia

Other causes, such as pericardial tamponade, myocardial infarction, bleeding, hemolysis, air embolism, or septicemia

Assessment of Biochemical Parameters

Blood Chemistries

The following laboratory tests should be monitored for the individual receiving chronic hemodialysis:

- BUN - this should be monitored at least monthly. Normal range is 7-20 mg/dL.
- Serum creatinine- monthly monitoring is recommended. Normal range is 0.5-1.5 mg/dL.
- Serum albumin- monthly monitoring. Target range is greater than 3.0 g/dL, and there is increased mortality risk for values lower than 3.0.
- Potassium- target value should be less than 5.0 mmol/L as this is associated with a lower mortality risk
- Phosphorus- should be measured monthly, and target range is less than 5.5 mg/dL for lowered mortality risk.
- Calcium- monthly monitoring is recommended, and target range is 8.4-10.2 mg/dL, (8.4-9.5 mg/dL for lowest mortality risk).
- Serum alkaline phosphatase- measure monthly and target value is less than 100 units/L. Mortality increases for levels greater than 150 units/L.

Clinical Significance of Laboratory Tests

- Blood urea nitrogen measures the amount of protein waste products found in the blood and is a measure of kidney function. This level is affected by protein intake.
- Serum creatinine is a measure of the waste products from muscle activity.
- Serum phosphorus measures how much phosphorus is in the blood and is important for preventing bone disease.
- Serum calcium measures how much calcium is in the blood and is important for preventing bone disease.
- Parathyroid hormone is affected by calcium and phosphorus levels and is important in preventing bone disease.
- Serum potassium measures how much potassium is in the blood and is directly affected by diet. Elevated potassium can affect muscle activity and heart function.
- Urine protein measures how much protein is in the urine and can indicate kidney damage if proteinuria continues.
- Urine albumin measures smaller particles of protein.
- Urine creatinine measures the amount of creatinine in the urine and is compared to the amount of albumin to indicate degree of kidney damage.
- Serum albumin measures the amount of albumin in the blood and is a measure of nutritional status.

- HDL cholesterol measures the amount of high density lipoprotein or good cholesterol in the blood to evaluate cardiac risk.
- LDL cholesterol measures low density lipoprotein or the bad cholesterol that may elevate cardiac risk.
- Serum triglycerides measure another type of fat that may also increase cardiac risk.

ANEMIA

The symptoms of anemia include decreased energy, increased fatigue or listlessness, trouble sleeping, inability to think clearly, shortness of breath, or a fast heart rate. Normal facial coloring may be paler than usual. Anemia can impact immune function. Kidneys normally produce erythropoietin (EPO) that stimulates red blood cell production. When kidney dysfunction is present, EPO is reduced, thus impairing red blood cell production. Anemia is more common in patients with diabetes, those who are African-American, or females. Individuals with Stage 3 or greater kidney failure will most likely develop anemia. Laboratory data that may be drawn to help diagnose or monitor anemia include hemoglobin, hematocrit, ferritin, and transferrin saturation.

ANEMIA IN INDIVIDUALS WITH CKD

For individuals with CKD and anemia, erythropoiesis-stimulating agents (ESA) are prescribed. These are usually given subcutaneously in the physician office. Additionally, supplemental iron is provided either orally or intravenously. The target value for hemoglobin is greater than 11 mg/dL according to the NKF K/DOQI guidelines. Consequences of untreated anemia may include the worsening of co-morbid conditions because of inadequate oxygen supply being delivered to tissues. This can also make the heart work harder and can lead to left ventricular hypertrophy (LVH). Many individuals with CKD develop LVH independent of anemia, but it is best to aggressively treat anemia when initially detected. Untreated anemia can also contribute to the patient feeling ill; once treated, the patient is likely to feel better and increase exercise. Treating anemia also reduces the risk of morbidity and mortality, and reduces admission to hospitals.

MONITORING ANEMIA

The tests used to diagnose and monitor for anemia include:

- Hemoglobin and hematocrit - hemoglobin should be greater than 11 g/dL in adults and greater than 11-12 g/dL in children. Hematocrit level should be greater than 33%.
- Serum ferritin and serum transferrin saturation (TSAT) - these are the most widely used for assessing iron status. Target values for adults are serum ferritin greater than 200 ng/dL and TSAT greater than 20%, according to the NKF K/DOQI guidelines. For children, serum ferritin should be greater than 100 ng/dL and TSAT should be greater than 20%

- Reticulocyte hemoglobin count (CHr) - this is a direct measure of available iron at the erythron level, thus it is a more sensitive and more cost-effective test than other tests. CHr should be greater than 29 pg/cell in adults; levels less than 29-32 pg/cell usually indicate iron deficiency.

eGFR

The estimated glomerular filtration rate (eGFR) is a way to estimate the level of kidney function. This validated equation used to calculate the eGFR is derived from the Modification of Diet in Renal Disease (MDRD) study. The equation is:

> eGFR (mL/min/1.73 m2) = 186 x (serum creatinine) – 1.154 x (age) – 0.203 x (0.742 if female) x (1.210 if African American).

It should be noted that serum creatinine does not increase above normal limits until greater than 50% of kidney function is lost. The National Kidney Foundation recommends that the eGFR be calculated each time a serum creatinine level is drawn to monitor kidney function in individuals who are at risk for developing CKD. The creatinine clearance test is no longer the preferred test for measuring kidney function because this test requires a 24-hour urine collection for creatinine. This is a cumbersome test with an opportunity for many mistakes to be made in the collection process. The eGFR is more cost effective and uses a lab value that is commonly checked during blood draws.

Factors That Influence eGFR and Serum Creatinine

The eGFR is affected by pregnancy. The eGFR should not be used for severely obese individuals, individuals with high or low amounts of muscle mass, very old or very young individuals, those with preexisting kidney disease as defined by proteinuria, and those whose renal function is greatly fluctuating on a daily basis such as those in acute renal failure. Individuals on any form of dialysis or with liver disease will likely have an unreliable result. Individuals who follow an alternative diet such as a strict vegetarian should be excluded. Additionally, those individuals who need the GFR measured because of renal clearance issues and medication use should be excluded. Instead, these individuals should have a measured GFR performed by a laboratory. Serum creatinine is used to monitor for trends in renal function; however, it is not sensitive enough on its own to monitor actual kidney function. Serum creatinine is affected by age, amount of muscle mass, and gender.

Serum Albumin

Serum albumin has long been used as a tool for assessing nutritional status. It is an indicator of visceral protein stores. This should be monitored every 3 months. Studies have shown serum albumin to be a good indicator of morbidity and mortality in individuals with CKD. A serum albumin concentration less than 4.0 g/dL has been associated with malnutrition in the CKD population. Levels less than 3.0 g/dL are at even higher risk for complications. Limitations of serum albumin include a relatively long half-life of approximately 20 days. Albumin is adversely affected by inflammation. Distribution of albumin in the intravascular and extracellular spaces may be affected by kidney disease. Serum albumin is also affected by proteinuria as well as losses in the dialysate. The presence of comorbid conditions such as diabetes or cardiovascular disease will affect albumin level as well as age.

Monitoring Bone Metabolism, Phosphorus and iPTH

All patients with chronic kidney disease (CKD) with a glomerular filtration rate (GFR) less than 60 mL/min/1.73 m2 should have serum calcium, phosphorus and intact parathyroid hormone (iPTH) levels monitored. The frequency is determined by the stage of kidney disease. For patients with stage 3 kidney disease, these labs should be monitored every 12 months. For patients with stage 4 kidney disease, these levels should be checked every 3 months. For patients with stage 5 kidney disease, serum calcium and phosphorus should be monitored every month, while iPTH should be monitored every 3 months. The target range for iPTH is as follows: stage 3, 35-70 pg/mL; stage 4, 70-110 pg/mL; and stage 5, 150-300 pg/mL. Patients with stage 3 or 4 CKD should have a serum phosphorus level maintained in the range of 2.7- 4.6 mg/dL, while patients with stage 5 or receiving dialysis should be maintained at a range of 3.5-5.5 mg/dL.

Target Range for Serum Calcium

Patients with stage 3 or 4 CKD should have serum calcium maintained within the normal range that the laboratory has defined. For patients with stage 5, maintaining serum calcium within normal limits or towards the lower end of the range, which is typically 8.4-9.5 mg/dL, is recommended. The serum calcium-phosphorus product is a measure used to predict the risk for the development of soft tissue calcification. This is important because it can lead to occlusion of the coronary arteries, thus increasing the risk for cardiovascular disease. This product should be maintained at less than 55 $mg^2/dL^2$for adolescents and adults and less than 65 mg^2/dL^2 for children. A product higher than this can lead to an increased risk of death. Total serum calcium levels need to be adjusted based on albumin level to more accurately reflect the free calcium level. The equation used to calculate this is as follows:

$$\text{Corrected calcium (mg/dL)} = \text{Total calcium (mg/dL)} + 0.08 \times [4 - \text{serum albumin (g/dL)}].$$

Dyslipidemia

According to the National Kidney Foundation's Kidney Disease Outcomes Quality Initiative (NKF K/DOQI), all adults and adolescents with CKD should be evaluated for the presence of dyslipidemia because of the increased risk for cardiovascular disease. This evaluation should include a fasting lipid panel consisting of total cholesterol, LDL and HDL level, and triglycerides. Those adolescents and adults with stage 5 CKD should be evaluated when diagnosed then should be monitored every 2-3 months if treatment changes, or at least annually.

Optimal target ranges for the fasting lipid panel should be as follows:

- Total cholesterol less than 200 mg/dL
- HDL cholesterol greater than 60 mg/dL for men and greater than 55 mg/dl for women
- LDL cholesterol less than 100 mg/dL
- Triglycerides less than 150 mg/dL

Definition of Dyslipidemia

Dyslipidemia as defined by the Adult Treatment Panel III (ATP III) is as follows:

- Total cholesterol less than 200 mg/dL is desirable, 200-230 mg/dL is borderline and greater than 240 mg/dL is considered high
- Low density lipoprotein (LDL) cholesterol less than 100 mg/dL is considered optimal, 100-129 is near optimal, 130-159 is borderline, 160-189 is high and greater than 190 is considered very high
- Triglycerides are considered to be normal at a level less than 150 mg/dL, 150-199 is borderline high, 200-499 is high and greater than 500 is very high.
- High density lipoprotein (HDL) levels should be greater than 40 mg/dL

Differences in the Guidelines for Managing Dyslipidemia

The NKF- K/DOQI and the NCEP ATP III guidelines for managing dyslipidemia in the CKD population are very similar but do have some key differences. The guidelines for the NKF- K/DOQI state that individuals with CKD should be treated as high risk, whereas the NCEP ATP III guidelines do not specify a different treatment plan for CKD patients, who are managed the same as the general population. The next difference is in how often dyslipidemia should be reevaluated. The NKF- K/DOQI guidelines state that reevaluation should occur after a change in health status or annually, whereas the NCEP ATP III states reevaluation every 5 years. Another key difference is when drug therapy should commence. The NKF- K/DOQI guidelines recommend starting drug therapy for an LDL level of 100-129 mg/dL after 3 months if therapeutic lifestyle changes have not been successful, whereas the NCEP ATP III guidelines state starting drug therapy is optional. Additionally, the first drug recommended by the NKF- K/DOQI is a statin, whereas NCEP ATP III guidelines give the option of 3 types of cholesterol- lowering agents.

NKF- K/DOQI for Children Recommendations

The NKF- K/DOQI guidelines differ slightly from those of the National Cholesterol Expert Panel on Children (NCEP-C). The NKF- K/DOQI guidelines recommend that adolescents with CKD be considered high risk and that a baseline evaluation of lipids should occur when CKD is diagnosed, then reevaluated with any change in treatment plans for kidney disease and also annually. Therapeutic lifestyle changes (TLC) should be implemented if LDL level is 130-159 mg/dL. After 6 months, a statin should be initiated if LDL level is still greater than 130 mg/dL. For an LDL level greater than 160 mg/dL, TLC should be started as well as a statin. The NCEP-C recommends that a drug therapy be initiated if LDL is greater than 160 mg/dL if there is a family history for heart disease and 2 or more additional risk factors are present. The NKF- K/DOQI guidelines are more intense and aimed to prevent the development of cerebrovascular disease.

Significance of the Presence of Dyslipidemia

Dyslipidemia plays a major role in the development of atherosclerotic cardiovascular disease. This is significant to the population with CKD because survival rates are poor due partly because of the co-morbid conditions of coronary heart disease, peripheral vascular disease, and cerebrovascular disease. The National Kidney Foundation (NKF) believes that there is a higher incidence of atherosclerotic cardiovascular disease in individuals with CKD and that individuals with CKD should be considered high risk for developing heart disease. The NKF Kidney Disease Outcomes Quality Initiative (K/DOQI) assembled a panel to address the management of dyslipidemia in patients with CKD. This included patients who had structural or functional issues with the kidney or who had a glomerular filtration rate (GFR) <60 mL/minute/1.73 m2 for a minimum of 3 months, as well as kidney transplant recipients.

Low Phosphorus Diet

There are several indications for initiating a dietary phosphorus restriction.

- For individuals with stage 3 or 4 CKD and a serum phosphorus level greater than 4.6 mg/dL, a dietary phosphorus restriction is indicated.
- A second indication is for any individual with renal failure with a serum phosphorus level greater than 5.5 mg/dL.
- A third indication is for individuals with an iPTH level that is above the target range for the appropriate stage of kidney disease.

Serum phosphorus is not typically adversely affected until the glomerular filtration rate falls to below 30 mL/min/1.73 m^2; however, secondary hyperparathyroidism may have started to develop, and serum phosphorus may not yet be elevated. Intervention is warranted. A restriction of 800-1000 mg per day of dietary phosphorus is the general recommendation. In individuals with stage 3 or 4 CKD, total dietary intake for elemental calcium should be limited to 2000 mg per day. This would include dietary sources as well as calcium supplements or calcium-based phosphate binders.

Hyperphosphatemia

The target range for phosphorus is 3.5-5.5 mg/dL for both hemodialysis and peritoneal dialysis patients. Hyperphosphatemia has been linked to cardiovascular issues and death. Keeping phosphorus within the target range will help to keep serum PTH within target range as well. Hyperphosphatemia will cause ionized calcium levels to decrease which in turn will stimulate PTH secretion. Hyperphosphatemia can be treated by a combination of methods. Restricting phosphorus intake to 800-1200 mg per day is recommended. Dialysis is also employed and will generally remove approximately 800 mg per dialysis session. Lastly, phosphorus binders are usually indicated. These products will bind phosphorus in the stomach, which prevents phosphorus from being absorbed. When prescribed as a phosphorus binder, this medication should be taken with meals.

UNA and TNA

TNA is also known as the protein equivalent of total nitrogen appearance and is used as a measure of protein intake and net protein breakdown for individuals receiving dialysis. It is most useful when a patient is in a steady state of nitrogen balance. It is less reliable for those who are in catabolic or anabolic stages such as pregnancy or growth. This calculation tries to take into account the many different ways that nitrogen can be lost, such as in urine, feces, or dialysate. The UNA is a way to measure net protein breakdown. The result of the UNA equation is then converted to total nitrogen appearance.

UNA (g/day) = Urinary Urea Nitrogen + blood urea nitrogen

= final serum urea nitrogen – initial serum urea nitrogen x 0.60 x initial body weight + (final body weight – initial body weight) x initial serum urea nitrogen

TNA (g/day) = 1.19 UNA + 1.27

The TNA can then be converted to protein equivalents by multiplying by 6.25.

Urea Kinetic Modeling

Urea kinetic modeling is a way to measure the adequacy of dialysis clearance by measuring how much blood was cleared of urea during the treatment compared to how much water was in a patient's body. This is an improved way of comparing the effect of treatment between patients of differing body weights and sizes. The basic equation is as follows:

$$Kt/v$$

Where "K" is the clearance of urea measured in mL/per minute, "t" is time measured in minutes and "v" is the amount of body water measured in liters. This equation utilizes pre- and post-dialysis blood urea nitrogen (BUN) values. The amount of protein that a patient is actually consuming is also calculated. Urea kinetic modeling can be calculated using the logarithm or by using specialized computer programs designed for this use.

Metabolic Acidosis and Metabolic Alkalosis

Metabolic acidosis is an excess of acid in the blood due to an alteration in the body's acid base balance. This may be caused by renal failure, diabetic ketoacidosis, or shock. It can also be caused by diarrhea, starvation, and certain medications. In metabolic acidosis, the pH level as well as the bicarbonate level will be low. Metabolic alkalosis is when there is too much bicarbonate in the blood. Because kidneys and lungs are responsible for regulating the amount of bicarbonate in the body, alterations in either of these organs can cause metabolic alkalosis. This can also be caused by the use of diuretics, vomiting, increased ingestion of an alkali, or an excessive loss of chloride. In metabolic alkalosis, both the pH and the bicarbonate level are increased.

Monitoring Children with Stage 2-4 CKD

Children with stage 2-4 chronic kidney disease (CKD) should have a serum 25-hydroxyvitamin D [25-(OH) D] level checked if the parathyroid hormone level is elevated. If the serum 25-(OH) D level is less than 30 ng/mL, a supplement of vitamin D in the form of ergocalciferol (vitamin D2) is indicated. Monitoring involves checking serum calcium and phosphorus monthly for 3 months, then every 3 months thereafter checking to see if levels are within normal limits. If serum calcium levels are greater than 10.2 mg/dL, then vitamin D supplements must be discontinued to decrease the risk of vitamin D toxicity. For children with elevated serum phosphorus levels, a restriction of dietary phosphorus should commence, but if this situation persists and the serum 25-(OH) D level is low, phosphate binders should be implemented to reduce the hyperphosphatemia, and vitamin D supplements should be continued. If in the previous scenario the 25- (OH) D level is normal, vitamin D supplements can be stopped.

Vitamin D Guidelines for Children

According to the NKF K/DOQI guidelines for children, vitamin D insufficiency should be diagnosed when the serum 25 hydroxyvitamin D [25 (OH) D] is between 16-30 ng/mL. Treatment should begin with 2000 international units of ergocalciferol everyday orally for 3 months. At this time, the serum 25 (OH) D level should be rechecked for improvement. Mild vitamin D deficiency is diagnosed when serum 25 (OH) D level is between 5-15 ng/mL. Treatment in this case should be 4000 international units of ergocalciferol orally per day for 3 months. The serum 25 (OH) D level should then be rechecked for improvement. A severe vitamin D deficiency is diagnosed when serum 25 (OH) D level is less than 5 ng/mL. Aggressive treatment is warranted starting with 8000 international units of ergocalciferol orally per day for 1 month followed by 4000 units per day orally for another 2 months with the serum level of 25 (OH) D rechecked at the end of the 3-month treatment.

Tight Glucose Control

Tight glucose control is difficult to attain in patients on dialysis primarily because of wide variations in food intake and food absorption, along with the overall impact of dialysis therapy. Poorly controlled diabetes increases the risk for all the complications of diabetes such as micro and macro vascular changes, cardiac disease, retinopathy, and all the other complications. There is a point in time where these changes are irreversible. When a patient is ready to start dialysis, many of the other changes are at the irreversible point. A value of less than 140 mg/dL is appropriate for fasting serum glucose and less than 200 mg/dL for postprandial serum glucose. The normal range for HgA1C is less than 7%, and patients receiving dialysis should strive to achieve a value as close to normal as possible.

Effect of Uremia on Insulin Metabolism

Uremia causes a decrease in insulin secretion from the beta cells of the pancreas. There is also a decrease in glucose uptake by peripheral tissues such as muscles. The half-life of insulin is extended in patients with uremia, and if the faster-acting type of insulin is used such as lispro, the onset of action is even faster than in patients without uremia, putting these patients at risk for hypoglycemia. The glucose tolerance test, which is often used to help diagnose diabetes, should not be utilized in patients receiving dialysis because of the insulin resistance associated with uremia. This will cause a longer, more sustained rise in blood glucose concentration. An elevated fasting glucose level in a patient without diabetes receiving hemodialysis may be indicative of diabetes. For those receiving peritoneal dialysis, a fasting glucose level cannot be checked due to a constant source of glucose in the dialysate solution. However, a level greater than 160 mg/dL may be indicative of diabetes.

Evaluation of Physical and Functional Status

Malnutrition

Individuals with CKD need to be continually monitored for the development of protein energy malnutrition. Possible indicators of malnutrition include:

- serum albumin less than 3.5 g/dL
- serum prealbumin less than 30 mg/dL
- low serum transferrin less than 200 mg/dL
- low serum creatinine despite worsening renal function
- actual body weight (dry weight, without the presence of edema) less than 85% of ideal weight
- loss of skinfold thickness, reduction of mid-arm muscle circumference (serial measures are helpful for assessing this)
- diet recall or evaluation of food diaries indicating suboptimal nutrient intake
- inadequate protein intake as evidenced by urea nitrogen excretion of less than 0.7 grams/kg per day

Factors That Contribute to Malnutrition or Wasting

There are many factors that contribute to the development of protein energy malnutrition (PEM) in patients with CKD. It should be noted that it is common to find the presence of PEM prior to the initiation of dialysis treatments. This may be attributed to hormonal changes, changes in protein and energy metabolism, or a deficiency in protein or calorie intake as kidney disease progresses. Once hemodialysis is initiated, patients receiving this mode of therapy long term are likely to develop PEM. This may be due to the procedure itself such as nutrient losses or inadequate therapy but there are other reasons as well. The presence of inflammation due to comorbidities such as diabetes, infections, dental problems, or cardiovascular disease may be the reason and this may cause anorexia or catabolism. Chronic metabolic acidosis may also be a cause. Disturbances in endocrine function such as elevated parathyroid hormone levels or insulin resistance are possible causes. Psychosocial issues that may be responsible for PEM include depression, financial issues, or lack of support system.

SGA

Subjective global assessment (SGA) is a clinical tool used for measuring nutritional status. It is especially useful for those patients receiving maintenance dialysis. This tool uses subjective and objective information obtained through medical history and physical examination. The history portion encompasses percent weight loss over a 6-month period; nutrient intake; the presence of certain GI symptoms such as anorexia, nausea, or vomiting; functional status; and metabolic issues related to co-morbid conditions. The physical exam portion evaluates the degree of subcutaneous fat, degree of temporal muscle wasting or wasting in the deltoids or quadriceps, presence of edema in the ankle or sacrum, and presence of ascites.

Evaluating Weight Change, Dietary Intake, the Severity of Gastrointestinal Symptoms, Degree of Subcutaneous Fat, and Muscle Wasting

Any practitioner such as a dietitian, nurse, or physician should be trained in performing a subjective global assessment (SGA). Weight change is evaluated by percentage of weight loss over a 6-month period with a less than 5% change indicating mild malnutrition, 5%-10% indicating moderate malnutrition, and a10% change indicating severe malnutrition. A subjective rating is then assigned based on a 7-point scale. If the weight change was planned, a lower score is assigned. Dietary intake is assessed by comparing actual intake to usual or recommended intake. A score based on the same 7-point scale is subjectively assigned to this as well. Subcutaneous fat is measured by looking at the fat pads below the patient's eyes and by checking the fat on the triceps and biceps. Muscle wasting is evaluated by looking at the temporal lobe area, the shoulders, visible presence of ribs or the scapula, and the muscle mass between the thumb and forefinger. Scores are assigned on the same 7-point scale for subcutaneous fat and muscle wasting. Higher scores indicate better nutritional status.

Weight

Weight should be obtained at roughly the same time, on the same scale and by the same practitioner if possible. Weight is most valuable when it is used as a trend over time to measure changes. For individuals with chronic kidney disease (CKD), a dry weight without the presence of edema or ascites should be used. This would account for metabolically active tissue only. Actual edema-free weight should be used if the weight is between 95%-115% of the median weight as defined by the National Health and Nutrition Examination Survey (NHANES II) data set. Adjusted edema-free body weight should otherwise be used. The equation to calculate this is as follows:

adjusted body weight (edema free) = actual edema-free body weight + [(standard body weight from NHANES II – body weight (edema free) x 0.25

This adjusted edema-free body weight should be used to calculate calorie and protein allowances.

Frame Size

One way of determining frame size is to measure elbow breadth. This information is then compared to data sets from National Health and Nutrition Examination Survey (NHANES I and II) that were published in the American Journal of Clinical Nutrition in 1984. Body composition is difficult to interpret. For example, an athlete may be considered overweight according to body mass index but in actuality, has a high degree of muscle mass. Body composition can be measured by the following:

- Triceps skin fold (TSF) measures the amount of body fat using skin fold calipers in the triceps, biceps, below the scapula, the upper thigh, and above the iliac crest.
- Mid-arm muscle circumference (MAMC) and mid-arm circumference (MAC) measure between the scapula and the elbow tip. It is a way to monitor for muscle wasting.
- Waist circumference measures around the waist below the ribs and above the belly button. This measures abdominal fat.
- Waist- to- hip ratio (WHR) measures the proportion of fat around the hips and waist.

Nutrition-Focused Physical Exam

A nutrition-focused physical exam is part of the nutrition assessment process that uses a systematic approach to evaluating a patient. The medical and nutritional history is utilized, as well as a physical exam. The main goal is to identify any possible nutrient deficiencies. The exam starts at the head and moves downward as data is gathered. The techniques used include:

- Inspection - this technique uses the senses (sight, smell, and hearing) to assess the patient
- Palpation - this technique assesses the texture, size, tenderness, etc., of certain body parts using the sense of touch
- Auscultation - uses hearing or a stethoscope to listen for different body sounds such as bowel sounds
- Percussion this technique uses tapping to assess sounds that reveal information about various organs

Abnormal Findings

General Observation

During a general observation or survey, the practitioner should be able to identify if an overt protein-calorie deficiency is present by observing muscle mass, fat stores, alterations in growth especially for children, and weight loss.

Skin

The exam of the skin would reveal possible issues with wound healing or the presence of decubitus ulcers that may indicate possible protein, vitamin C, or zinc deficiency. It may also reveal excessive fat stores that may indicate excess calorie consumption. The skin may also reveal dryness or scaly textures indicative of possible vitamin A or essential fatty acid deficiency. Skin that is excessively pale may indicate an iron or folic acid deficiency. Dermatitis or red skin lesions could indicate possible niacin deficiency. Excessive bruising or petechiae may indicate vitamin K or C deficiency. If the skin has a yellowish pigment, it could be due to excessive carotene intake.

Scalp, Hair, Nails or Eyes

Abnormalities in the scalp such as softening or an open anterior fontanel in a child may indicate possible vitamin D deficiency. Hair that is thin and falling out or has lost its shine may indicate a possible protein or zinc deficiency. Spoon-shaped nails can be indicative of an iron deficiency. Nails that are pale or blotchy may indicate vitamin A or C deficiency. If the eyes have pale conjunctiva, a deficiency of iron, folate, or vitamin B12 may be responsible. A vitamin A deficiency can manifest with night blindness, Bitot's spots (yellow or white foamy type spots on the whites of the eyes), cornea that appear milky in nature, whites of the eyes and the inner eyelid that appear dry and rough, or softening of the cornea. Eyes that are red and cracked in the corners may indicate riboflavin or niacin deficiency.

Lips, Mouth, Tongue, Gums, Teeth

Abnormalities in the area of the lips of mouth such as cracking and redness of the lips may be due to a deficiency of riboflavin, niacin, or pyridoxine. Cheilosis, which means scaling, inflammation, or reddening of the lips or fissures in the corners of the mouth, can be caused by riboflavin or niacin deficiency. A tongue that is magenta in color may be due to a riboflavin deficiency. A tongue that is red and swollen or smooth and slick may be indicative of riboflavin, folate, niacin, or B12 deficiency. Decreased taste acuity may be a result of a zinc deficiency. Gums that are bleeding and spongy can indicate a deficiency of vitamin C. Teeth that are mottled may indicate excessive fluoride, or teeth in general poor condition with cavities may indicate an excessive intake of sugar or sugary foods.

Chest/Lungs, Heart, Kidneys

Abnormal findings in the chest/lung such as fat wasting or somatic muscle wasting may indicate protein calorie malnutrition. Changes in respiratory status such as difficult or labored breathing or rapid breathing may indicate a possible metabolic acidosis or metabolic alkalosis. In terms of cardiac issues, irregular rhythm may be due to a deficiency of potassium, calcium, or magnesium, or a severe deficiency of phosphorus. Fluid status can affect the activity of the pulse. A fast pulse may indicate fluid overload, while a slow and weak pulse may indicate dehydration. A deficiency of thiamin can cause tachycardia and an enlarged heart. The kidney, ureter, and bladder can also indicate fluid status by the condition of the urine. Concentrated urine or a decrease in urine output can indicate dehydration.

Musculoskeletal and Neurologic

Protein calorie malnutrition may be seen in the musculoskeletal system by wasting in the arms or legs, swelling of the joints, or a decrease in the range of motion. Vitamin C deficiency can also be observed with swollen and tender joints. If bowed legs are present, vitamin D or calcium deficiency should be suspected. If the epiphyses of the long bones including the wrists, knees, or ankles are enlarged, this could indicate a possible vitamin C or D deficiency. In terms of the neurological exam, changes in psychomotor activity, confusion, or peripheral neuropathy may be a result of a deficiency of vitamin B12, thiamin, pyridoxine, and possibly protein. If hyperactive reflexes are present, a calcium deficiency may be the cause. The presence of tetany, which is spasms of the voluntary muscles, may be due to a calcium or magnesium deficiency. General observation during mealtime indicating decreased mental acuity or inability to efficiently feed oneself may help to evaluate the individual's overall nutritional status.

Relation of Nutrients to Skin Integrity

Water, Vitamin A, Vitamin C, Vitamin E and Vitamin K

Nutrition is one of the major factors that impact skin integrity. Water is extremely important as it maintains hydration and keeps skin feeling fresh and healthy. Water helps to remove toxins and helps to transport vitamins, minerals, and oxygen to cells. The anti-oxidant vitamin A helps to maintain healthy skin and improves the elasticity of the skin. Vitamin C is needed for collagen production and for the growth and repair of tissues throughout the body. It is also required for wound healing. Vitamin E, another anti-oxidant, helps to protect the body from damage by free radicals and helps with skin integrity. Vitamin K helps with blood clotting, and a deficiency in this vitamin may cause bruising or bleeding.

Vitamin B Complex, Zinc, Copper, Omega 3 Fatty Acids

The B complex vitamins play an important role in skin integrity. A deficiency of niacin can cause dermatitis. Both vitamin B6 and B12 play a role in red blood cell production. Biotin is necessary for protein synthesis. Folate helps with red blood cell production as well as the production of DNA, which regulates tissue growth. Zinc is required for collagen production as well as wound healing. A deficiency of zinc can manifest in skin conditions such as dermatitis. Copper is needed for the production of collagen as well as maintaining the elasticity of skin. Omega 3 fatty acids help to protect the skin from ultraviolet light. They also prevent essential fatty acid deficiency.

Fluid Status in Hemodialysis or Peritoneal Dialysis

There are many factors that affect fluid status in patients receiving either hemodialysis or peritoneal dialysis. One factor may be noncompliance with fluid and/or sodium restriction. Another factor may be loss of residual renal function or inadequate dialysis runs. For peritoneal dialysis patients, fluid overload may be due to selecting the wrong type of solution (i.e., a lower dextrose concentration). Fluid overload may also be due to an abdominal leak, or mechanical issues, such as catheter malfunction, or issues with the peritoneal membrane performance. Volume status and blood pressure should be closely monitored for all patients receiving dialysis to ensure euvolemia.

Nutritional Parameters for Children over the Age of 2 with CKD

The general opinion of the National Kidney Foundation K/DOQI guidelines favors monitoring of most of the following parameters every 3-4 months. The exceptions are serum albumin and bicarbonate, which should be measured every month. These may be done more frequently as needed based on the child's progress. The parameters that should be monitored include:

- Standing height and height for chronological age
- Estimation of dry weight. Weight should be measured in light clothing and measured to the nearest 0.1 kg
- Head circumference until the age of 36 months
- Weight for height index and Z scores
- Skinfold thickness and mid-arm muscle circumference
- Dietary interview
- Urea kinetic modeling

Psychosocial Issues

There are a myriad of psychosocial issues that may affect the individual with CKD. Depression is one of the most common problems. This condition may be under-reported and as a result, under-treated. This may lead to noncompliance with the medical treatment plan, including medication use, dialysis, and adherence to dietary restrictions. It sometimes can lead to suicide. Screening for depression is essential in this population. Deficits in brain function can also be observed in the form of dementia or delirium. This may be due to uremia or other co-morbid conditions. Anxiety or other behavioral issues are present at times and should be addressed. Marital conflict can be seen at times and may be due to the way the patient views his or her illness, its burden on others (especially the spouse), and how well the patient is complying with the treatment plan. There is a high rate of sexual dysfunction that can also play a role in marital issues. Financial issues are a possibility, as many dialysis patients are not able to work when dialysis begins.

Evaluation of Medicine & Supplements

Phosphorus Binder

Phosphorus binders are indicated as an adjunct to a dietary phosphorus restriction when the restriction alone is not enough to reduce serum phosphorus and/or parathyroid hormone level. Phosphorus binders may also be used if further restriction of dietary phosphorus intake will compromise other required nutrients. There are many different types of phosphorus binders, and the choice on which to use is individual to each patient. Sometimes a combination of medications is required, and this may help to reduce the amount of side effects a patient may experience from using only one form of therapy, such as hypercalcemia with the sole use of a calcium-containing phosphorus binder. The choice of therapy also depends on the patient's willingness to comply with therapy. The mechanism for phosphorus binders is that they bind phosphorus in the gut, thus preventing absorption. Phosphorus binders should be taken with meals.

Calcium Carbonate and Magnesium Carbonate

Calcium carbonate binders are available as TUMS, Os-Cal and Caltrate, Calcichew and Titralac. This type of binder is available in multiple doses ranging from 500 mg to 1250 mg. 40% of the dose is considered to be elemental calcium. Calcium intake from binders should not exceed 1500 mg of elemental calcium per day, and total calcium intake from binders and diet should not exceed 2000 mg per day. This type of binder is relatively inexpensive and available over the counter. Possible side effects of this type of binder include constipation, hypercalcemia, or extra-skeletal calcification. Magnesium carbonate binders are available as MagneBind 200 that contains 200 mg MgCO3 with 400 mg CaCO3 and MagneBind 300 that contains 300 mg MgCO3 and 250 CaCO3. 40% of the calcium dose is considered elemental. Possible side effects of this type of binder include elevated serum magnesium level and diarrhea.

Calcium Acetate, Sevelamer Hydrochloride, and Lanthanum Carbonate

Calcium acetate binders are available as PhosLo or Calphron and contain 169 mg elemental calcium per tablet. There is less calcium absorption than with the calcium carbonate form of binders, and these are more expensive and require a prescription. Possible side effects include hypercalcemia, nausea, vomiting, or constipation. Sevelamer hydrochloride is available as Renagel. This product is available as 400- and 800-mg tablets. It does not contain any calcium and is aluminum-free. It is especially helpful for patients who are prone to developing hypercalcemia. It is more expensive than other phosphorus binding therapies, and multiple pills are often required to achieve phosphorus control. It acts as a bile salt binder and has the added benefit of lowering LDL levels. Possible side effects include nausea, vomiting, and diarrhea. Hypocalcemia is also possible. Lanthanum carbonate is available as Fosrenol. It is a chewable product and is expensive. It is also calcium- and aluminum-free. Possible side effects include nausea, vomiting, and diarrhea.

Aluminum-Based Binders

Aluminum hydroxide binders are available as AlternaGEL, Alu-Cap, or Amphojel. Aluminum carbonate binders are available as Basagel. These types of binders were popular in the 1980's but are not considered to be primary therapy due to the potential for aluminum toxicity. These may be used for a short time if serum phosphorus is severely elevated greater than 7.0 mg/dL or if the calcium x phosphate product is severely elevated in a patient with hyperparathyroidism. Short term is defined as less than 4 weeks. Possible side effects of aluminum-based binders include severe constipation or fecal impaction, chalky taste, nausea, vomiting, and abdominal discomfort.

Calcitriol in Children with CKD

For children with stage 2-4 CKD, calcitriol should be initiated when parathyroid hormone (PTH) levels are greater than the target range as defined by the actual stage of CKD, and if serum 25 hydroxyvitamin D levels are greater than 30 ng/mL. Caution should be taken that serum calcium levels are not elevated and serum phosphorus levels are within normal limits, and these levels should be monitored monthly. PTH level should be rechecked every 3 months. If a decrease in PTH is achieved to within the appropriate target range, calcitriol should be held. If serum calcium levels are greater than 10.2 mg/dL, calcitriol should be held to avoid the possibility of vitamin D toxicity. If PTH level does not respond appropriately with at least a 30% reduction and serum calcium and phosphorus levels are in the appropriate range, the calcitriol dose should be increased by 50%. Serum PTH, calcium, and phosphorus should then be measured every month for 3 months.

Calcitriol Initiated in Children Receiving Hemodialysis

An elevated serum parathyroid hormone (PTH) level greater a child with stage 5 kidney disease receiving hemodialysis warrants immediate initiation of calcitriol. Parameters that should also be monitored include serum calcium, phosphorus, and the calcium x phosphate product. These parameters should be serum calcium less than 10 mg/dL, serum phosphorus less than 6.5 mg/dL for adolescents or less than 5.5 for children younger than 12 years of age, calcium x phosphate product less than 55 for children younger than 12 or less than 65 for children older than 12 for the appropriate initiation of calcitriol. For the above parameters and:

- PTH between 300-500 pg/mL, calcitriol should be initiated at 0.0075 μg/kg per day.
- PTH greater than 500-1000 pg/mL, calcitriol should be initiated at 0.015 μg/kg per day.
- PTH greater than 1000 pg/mL, calcitriol should be initiated at 0.025 μg/kg per day.

Vitamin D Analogs Calcitriol and Doxercalciferol

Commonly used forms of vitamin D analogs include:

- Calcitriol [1, 25-(OH) 2 D2] - this is known under the trade name as Rocaltrol for the oral route and Calcijex as the IV route. The starting dose for the oral form is 0.25 micrograms per day and the IV form is 0.02 micrograms per kg three times per week usually given during hemodialysis. Side effects are not common with this medication but may include headache, feeling tired, nausea, or vomiting. Serum calcium and phosphorus should be checked every month.
- Doxercalciferol – this medication is a vitamin D prohormone that will convert in the liver to the active form of vitamin D [1, 25-(OH) 2 D2]. Hectorol is the trade name for both the oral and IV form of the medication. The starting dose for both forms is 2.5-5 micrograms three times per week. It is used for patients with stage 5 chronic kidney disease (CKD) on dialysis with elevated parathyroid hormone (PTH) levels or for stage 3-4 CKD not on dialysis with elevated PTH. Side effects may include swelling, headaches, general malaise, or shortness of breath.

Vitamin D Analogs Paricalcitol

Paricalcitol is a vitamin D analog that has been shown to be not as effective as other vitamin D analogs in treating hyperparathyroidism despite its success in animals. It has also not been studied for use in patients under the age of 18 or older than 65. This is available as Zemplar for both the oral and IV forms of the drug. The starting dose for the oral form is 1-2 micrograms per day or 2-4 micrograms per week. For the IV form, the starting dose is 0.04-0.1 microgram/kg. Possible side effects include chills, general malaise, tachycardia, vomiting, dry mouth, or nausea and vomiting.

Heparin

There is a risk of bleeding for patients on heparin, especially for those who have gastritis, peptic ulcer disease, or have had a recent surgery. There is also a risk of hypertriglyceridemia. This may occur because of the activation of lipoprotein lipase by heparin. Heparin can also lower the levels of HDL cholesterol. There is also a risk of developing heparin-associated thrombocytopenia due to either a decrease in platelet count related to heparin dose and timing, or the development of certain antibodies that act against the heparin platelet factor. Heparin can also cause pruritus or itching possibly due to an allergic reaction. Hyperkalemia is also a possibility due to the suppression of aldosterone synthesis by heparin. Low molecular weight heparin may be useful in preventing hyperkalemia as well as lipid alterations and itching, but should not be used for treating heparin-induced thrombocytopenia.

Insulin Regimen

It is advisable for initial insulin doses to be reduced by 25%-50% in patients with diabetes who also receive hemodialysis. This is because of the longer half-life of insulin due to uremic conditions. Insulin itself is not removed by the hemodialysis process. The use of long-acting insulin divided into two doses with supplementation by short-acting insulin at mealtime is one way to attain reasonable glucose control. For patients with diabetes receiving peritoneal dialysis, insulin can be given either subcutaneously or via the dialysis solution. Receiving the insulin dose via the dialysate enables tighter glucose control because the dose can be adjusted based on glucose level. Additionally, the dose can be based on the type of dextrose concentration being given as part of the dialysate. Care must be taken to make sure the insulin mixes with the dialysate, and a long needle should be utilized to administer the insulin all the way into the bag. Typically, the dose added to the dialysate is 2-3 times above the normal subcutaneous dose. Close glucose monitoring is essential.

Oral Hypoglycemic Agents

The majority of oral hypoglycemic agents have not been studied for use in patients receiving dialysis. Some agents can be used but require close monitoring and supervision. Metformin is one agent that should be avoided for those receiving dialysis. This drug has been shown to cause lactic acidosis and has reduced renal clearance. Glyburide is another agent that should be avoided because it may cause hypoglycemia in patients receiving dialysis because of impaired renal excretion of the drug. Alpha-glucosidase inhibitors such as Acarbose or Miglitol should be avoided because of the type of mechanism involved. Sulfonylureas such as Glipizide, Glimepiride, and Tolbutamide are probably the safest choices if oral hypoglycemic agents are required. These medications have a shorter half-life and are metabolized mainly in the liver.

Anemia

Anemia of CKD is caused by inadequate production of erythropoietin (EPO) in the renal tubules. As renal function worsens, there is concomitant reduction in EPO, and anemia gradually develops. The main type of medication used to treat anemia of CKD is recombinant human erythropoietin referred to as erythropoiesis-stimulating agents (ESAs). The brand names that are available include Epogen, Procrit, and Aranesp. ESA should be started when hemoglobin levels fall below 10 g/dL. The current recommendation for appropriate hemoglobin level by the NKF K/DOQI guidelines is 11 g/dL for adults and 11-12 g/dL for children. ESA can be given subcutaneously or intravenously. The intravenous route is the most commonly used route for hemodialysis patients most likely because of the discomfort associated with subcutaneous injections.

Anemia Treatment

Patients should be educated on the benefits of anemia treatment. These include the following:

- Reduced mortality risk - studies have demonstrated an increase in death for patients with hemoglobin levels less than 10 g/dL. This risk begins to decrease once hemoglobin levels are above 11 g/dL

- Decreased frequency of hospitalization and decreased length of stay for individuals with hemoglobin levels greater than 11 g/dL
- Reduced need for transfusions
- Improved bleeding time
- Improvement in overall quality of life related to feeling less tired, with an increase in ability to exercise and get around more. If pruritus is present, the itching may be relieved with therapy
- Improved mental capacity in terms of ability to focus and be attentive
- Possibility that left ventricular hypertrophy may improve

Treatment of Anemia Using Oral Iron Supplements

Oral iron supplements used to treat anemia in dialysis patients is associated with less than desirable outcomes. Oral iron supplements may also cause gastrointestinal side effects such as constipation, diarrhea, or excessive gas. Oral iron is not recommended for hemodialysis patients because studies have not shown any improved outcomes using oral iron. For those patients receiving peritoneal dialysis, ferrous sulfate may be used as well as ferrous fumarate or ferrous gluconate. 200 mg of elemental iron per day for adults and 2-3 mg/kg up to 6 mg/kg for children is the recommended dosage. Oral iron should be provided on an empty stomach to promote the best absorption possible and should not be taken at the same time as phosphate binders. Side effects may be minimized by giving the dose at bedtime or during dialysis sessions, or by giving smaller doses to minimize the iron load delivered to the duodenum at one time. Aggressively treating constipation using laxatives or stool softeners is also recommended.

ESA Therapy

Side Effects

The main potential side effect of erythropoiesis-stimulating agent (ESA) therapy is the need for increased doses of antihypertensive drugs because of unstable hypertension as anemia is corrected. This may occur in up to one third of dialysis patients. Other potential side effects include seizures related to a quick rise in hemoglobin level. There is also a risk of graft clotting as blood becomes thicker with improvement in anemia. There may also be a reduction in urea clearance with improvement in hemoglobin levels due to a lower ratio of plasma to red cell volume. Occasional hyperkalemia is experienced. Phosphorus levels may be more difficult to control. This may be related to a better appetite and possible increased phosphorus intake as a result, along with a reduction in phosphorus clearance as hemoglobin levels improve.

Effect of Iron Deficiency

Iron deficiency can cause a poor response to ESA therapy. This is because iron is required to produce red blood cells and must be available for ESA therapy to be effective. Iron deficiency may be due to a number of reasons:

- Chronic blood loss due to the hemodialysis process itself, blood draws for laboratory work, gastrointestinal bleeding, or bleeding from the access site.
- Increased demands due to ESA therapy (called functional iron deficiency)
- Decreased iron absorption related to phosphate binder therapy or medications used to treat gastrointestinal distress such as H2 blockers or proton pump inhibitors
- Decreased absorption related to uremia

IV Iron Therapy

Hemodialysis Patients

IV iron is commonly used to treat iron deficiency in hemodialysis patients because it improves iron availability and utilization. Improvement in anemia is more easily achieved using IV iron compared to oral iron supplements. There are 3 types that may be used: iron dextran, ferric gluconate, and iron sucrose. There are two options for adult dosing. The first is to provide 1000 mg over the course of 8-10 hemodialysis sessions. The other option is to assume that iron deficiency will be chronic and provide a maintenance dose of 25-100 mg per week. For children, 1-2 mg/kg per week of elemental iron should be provided. It should be noted that IV iron is more expensive than the oral form.

Safety of IV Iron

The first potential safety issue with intravenous IV iron is the risk for anaphylaxis with iron dextran. It is a rare occurrence and is very dangerous. The signs of anaphylaxis include rapid onset of symptoms, hypotension, difficulty breathing, flushing of the face, and pain in the back. Typically, a test dose is given, and the patient is closely monitored for signs of reaction. A second safety issue is the risk for infection because iron provides an optimal environment for the growth of bacteria. It is recommended that iron therapy be avoided during times of infection to minimize risk of complications. A third safety issue is the potential for oxidation. Because iron is an oxidative substance, it has the potential to cause oxidative damage to certain types of proteins. It may also cause an exacerbation of vascular oxidation that may cause atherosclerotic damage. Lastly, there is potential for iron overload leading to oxidative stress at the cellular level.

Dialysis Patients

Multivitamins Available

There are many types of multivitamin preparations available for use with patients receiving hemodialysis. These patients are at risk for developing vitamin deficiencies especially water-soluble vitamins. The brand names that are available include Nephrocaps, Renal Tab, and Dialyvite 800 with zinc, Diatx, and Renax. These multivitamin preparations are specially formulated to address the concerns of deficiencies and potential toxicities for dialysis patients. Vitamin A is not included due to risk for toxicity and this may affect bone resorption. Folic acid is added in higher amounts to cover losses in the dialysate and to help prevent elevated homocysteine levels that have been linked to cardiovascular disease. Additional B vitamins are provided as well to cover losses in dialysate. Vitamin C is provided at 75-90 mg at levels that will not cause increased oxalate levels. Zinc is included in certain preparations, as is selenium.

Carnitine Supplementation

Carnitine is an amino acid that has a role in fat metabolism and energy production. There is evidence that L-carnitine levels are suboptimal in patients receiving dialysis. Symptoms of carnitine deficiency may include anemia, skeletal muscle weakness, cardiomyopathy, and encephalopathy. The routine use of supplemental L-carnitine in dialysis patients remains controversial. Some studies have suggested a role for dialysis patients with anemia, intradialytic hypotension, and cardiomyopathy. The NKF K/DOQI guidelines do not recommend routine supplementation until further randomized controlled studies have been completed. L-carnitine may be prescribed for a documented L-carnitine deficiency as evidenced by a plasma-free carnitine level less than 40 µmol/L. Dosing is generally 20 mg/kg administered intravenously at the end of the dialysis session.

rhGH for Children

Growth in childhood can be severely affected by chronic kidney disease and maintenance dialysis. A child should be considered for treatment with recombinant human growth hormone (rhGH) if certain criteria are met. These criteria include a child whose height for chronological age is more than 2 standard deviation scores below standard, whose height velocity growth for chronological age is more than 2 standard deviation scores below the standard, who has evidence of being able to achieve growth potential because of an open epiphyses, and who should not have any contraindications to therapy. The contraindications that must be addressed before therapy can begin include the achievement and maintenance of adequate nutrient intake including calories and protein in order to optimize growth, correction of acidosis, correction of hyperphosphatemia, and correction of hyperparathyroidism. If a child does not respond to treatment with rhGH within 12 months, suspension of treatment should be considered. A good response to treatment would be an increase of at least 2 cm in height.

Kidney Transplant Patients

Cyclosporine A

Immunosuppressive therapy is initiated in the immediate post-transplant period to help prevent rejection of the transplanted organ. Cyclosporine A, known by the trade names of Sandimmune or Neoral, can have significant nutritional implications. Laboratory abnormalities are a possibility including hyperkalemia, hyperglycemia, and hypomagnesemia. A potassium restriction may be indicated to reduce serum potassium. A controlled carbohydrate diet may be indicated to address hyperglycemia, and magnesium supplements may be indicated to normalize serum magnesium. Cyclosporine A can also cause hyperplasia in the mouth, which can be addressed with good oral hygiene. GI distress such as nausea, vomiting, or loss of appetite is possible, which can be addressed with individualized counseling with the dietitian. The patient may require a modified diet or nutritional supplements. Lastly, hyperlipidemia is possible and a therapeutic lifestyle change (TLC) diet should be implemented.

Azathioprine

Azathioprine is also known by the trade name of Imuran. It is prescribed to help prevent organ rejection in patients who have had kidney transplants. The main side effects of this drug are nausea, vomiting, abdominal distress, diarrhea, and muscle aches and pains. This drug can also cause cholestasis of the liver. For the GI complaints, a modified diet or temporary liquid diet may help or the addition of nutritional supplements may be required. Other side effects may include ulcerations of the mouth, which may be painful when eating. A texture-modified diet with supplements may be helpful. Other potential side effects include lethargy, decreased appetite, and infection. If an infection occurs, additional calories may be required to compensate.

Corticosteroids

Corticosteroids are immunosuppressants used for kidney transplant patients to help prevent rejection of the transplanted organ and provide anti-inflammatory protection. They are also known as glucocorticoids, and the drugs commonly prescribed are prednisone or methylprednisolone. Side effects can include impaired wound healing and an increase in protein catabolism, both of which require an increase in protein intake. Other side effects can include hyperglycemia that can lead to steroid-induced diabetes. A controlled carbohydrate diet and other usual diet modifications will be indicated in this case. Corticosteroids can also affect lipid levels and cause an increase in appetite, which often leads to weight gain. Potential for weight gain and increased lipid levels need to be addressed when educating the patient about potential side effects of this drug. This type of drug has major implications for bones, and the patient should be monitored closely. Children may experience changes in growth. Other side effects may include increased fatigue, muscle aches, and heartburn. There are many other side effects to this medication that are not directly related to nutrition.

Tacrolimus

Tacrolimus is one of the newer drugs used for immunosuppression following kidney transplant. It is known by the trade name Prograf or FK506. This drug may cause hypertension, and a sodium-restricted diet may need to be implemented. Tacrolimus can also cause hyperglycemia. A carbohydrate-controlled diet should be instituted to help manage blood glucose levels, and simple sugars should be restricted. Hyperkalemia is also a possibility and may require restriction of dietary potassium. Tacrolimus may cause GI side effects such as nausea, vomiting, diarrhea, abdominal pain, and decreased appetite. The patient should work closely with the dietitian to find foods he or she can tolerate. Nutritional supplements may be indicated. This drug can also cause weight gain or swelling in the extremities. The patient should be monitored closely and may require sodium restriction for swelling or tips on weight control if unplanned weight gain is occurring.

CKD Patients

Anorexia

Anorexia is a commonly seen issue in patients with end stage renal disease. Dietary intervention with a registered dietitian should be attempted before medication is prescribed. If medication is required, two choices include Megestrol and Dronabinol. Megestrol is known by the trade name of Megace and may cause gastrointestinal side effects such as diarrhea or constipation, heartburn, nausea, or vomiting. It can also cause an increase in thirst and frequency of urination. Other side effects can include weakness, pain, or numbness in the extremities. Dronabinol is known by the trade name of Marinol. It is an appetite stimulant and anti-emetic that can be habit forming. It can cause side effects that involve the central nervous system, such as mood changes, anxiety, hallucinations, memory loss, or confusion. This drug can cause alterations in sleep habits once the drug is stopped. It can also cause tachycardia and seizures.

Factors Contributing to Anorexia, Nausea, and Vomiting

Anorexia is typically a symptom associated with uremia; however, there are other causes such as infection that should be fully evaluated. Uremia causes anorexia because as renal function declines, nitrogenous waste products build up in the blood producing these symptoms. A person who has not been dialyzed adequately may experience anorexia until the dialysis is adjusted. Other factors that may contribute to anorexia include other co-morbid conditions and certain medications. Before dialysis has been established as a therapy, many individuals may also experience nausea and vomiting. Once the uremia has been cleared through dialysis, symptoms should be alleviated. If nausea and vomiting continue, further investigation is warranted.

Dyspepsia

Dyspepsia, commonly known as indigestion, is defined as pain in the upper abdominal area that can be described as burning or gaseous. The symptoms include abdominal discomfort, bloating and gassy feeling accompanied by burping or flatulence. There are many causes of dyspepsia. The most common causes can be peptic ulcer disease (PUD), gastroesophageal reflux disease (GERD), gastritis or duodenitis. For individuals with diabetes, it can be caused by gastroparesis. In individuals receiving dialysis, dyspepsia can be caused by certain medications, most notably iron supplements and phosphate binders. The most common medications used to treat dyspepsia for these individuals are prokinetic agents, proton pump inhibitors such as esomeprazole (Nexium), omeprazole (Prilosec), lansoprazole (Prevacid) or pantoprazole (Protonix), and histamine-2 blockers such as cimetidine (Tagamet), ranitidine (Zantac), famotidine (Pepcid), or nizatidine (Axid).

Constipation

Constipation in individuals with renal failure has a number of possible causes. One is decreased fluid intake especially for those who are pre-dialysis or for those receiving hemodialysis. Another cause may be the avoidance of certain fruits and vegetables that may contribute to potassium intake thus reducing dietary fiber intake. Certain medications may also contribute to constipation, including iron supplements and calcium-based phosphate binders. The use of narcotics such as codeine or morphine can contribute to constipation, and decreased physical activity can also be a factor. Possible consequences of untreated constipation are obstipation and obstruction, fecal impaction, and in some cases, perforation of the bowel. Constipation can also lead to diverticular disease due to attempts to move the bowel and increased intracolonic pressures, both of which can lead to herniations in the colon. Constipation can also cause hemorrhoids. For individuals receiving peritoneal dialysis, chronic constipation can block the outflow of the dialysate leading to additional issues.

Treatments for Constipation

Dietary intervention is the first step in treating constipation. This involves increasing fiber intake slowly over the course of 2-3 weeks. Increasing fluid intake is also beneficial but may not be medically appropriate for many renal patients. Medications may also be prescribed such as docusate sodium (Colace), which is an emollient; bisacodyl (Dulcolax), which is a stimulant; or lactulose (Chronulac) or polyethylene glycol (Miralax), which are both hyperosmotics. Enemas or glycerin suppositories may also be given for quicker results. Phosphate-containing enemas should be avoided as they can cause dangerous complications such as hyperphosphatemia, hypocalcemia, or rectal necrosis. Increasing physical activity to the best of the patient's ability is also recommended as a way to alleviate constipation.

Contraindicated Treatments for Constipation

The use of sodium polystyrene sulfonate and sorbitol (Kayexalate) in the treatment of constipation is not advisable in patients with end stage renal disease (ESRD) because it may cause intestinal necrosis. Additionally, psyllium-based medication such as Metamucil should not be used as a treatment for constipation in patients with kidney failure. The reason for this is that it contains high amounts of sodium and potassium, and it requires a large amount of fluid to prepare. Laxatives should also be avoided in patients with ESRD. Those that contain magnesium can cause high levels of magnesium to build up in the blood due to poor clearance of magnesium by the kidneys. This can lead to bradycardia or the development of neurologic problems. Citrate-containing laxatives should also be avoided because citrate increases aluminum absorption in the gut. This can lead to aluminum toxicity that can cause neurological symptoms such as confusion, agitation or seizures, or osteomalacia. Examples of products to be avoided include milk of magnesia, Fleet's products, and magnesium citrate.

Diarrhea

Possible causes of diarrhea in patients with ESRD are usually similar to causes in individuals without ESRD. A common cause may be related to changes in diet, changes in fiber intake or as a result of viral infection. Unresolved diarrhea may be due to inflammatory bowel disease and an endoscopy may be warranted for diagnostic purposes. Diarrhea as a result of an infection is usually accompanied by a fever. In this case, stool cultures should be obtained to determine the cause. Many patients may develop *Clostridioides difficile* infection following a lengthy course of antibiotics. Malabsorption is also a possibility, especially if fat or fibrous matter is visible in the stool. If the diarrhea is bloody and is accompanied by pain in the abdomen, fever, and a drop in blood pressure, then an ischemic origin may be possible and immediate medical attention is imperative. This may be a result of a bowel perforation.

Treatment Options for Noninfectious Diarrhea

Noninfectious diarrhea in a patient with ESRD can be treated in different ways. Certain medications, such as attapulgite (Kaopectate), diphenoylate hydrochloride and atropine sulfate (Lomotil), and loperamide hydrochloride (Imodium), can safely be used in patients with ESRD. Changes in diet can also help. Adding fiber can help to slow transit time in the gut but care must be taken to consume foods that fit within the individual diet restrictions, such as potassium. Lactose can be avoided if lactase deficiency is suspected or if the patient has been on long-term antibiotics. Probiotics are sometimes used to help replenish or change the bacteria in the gut; however, the use of probiotics has not been specifically studied in patients with ESRD, although research studies are currently getting underway in this area.

Upper GI Bleeding

Possible causes of upper gastrointestinal GI bleeding in patients with CKD include duodenal ulcers, erosive gastritis, duodenitis, esophagitis, or a Mallory-Weis tear. The cause of bleeding is typically determined via esophagogastroduodenoscopy (EGD). The presence of *Helicobacter pylori* may be the origin of gastritis or peptic ulcer disease. This is generally treated with a combination of antibiotics and proton pump inhibitors. Care should be taken with dosing of medications in CKD. Otherwise, upper GI bleeding is treated in the same way as it is in patients without CKD. An acid secretion inhibitor, proton pump inhibitor, or histamine-2 blocker can be used. Histamine-2 blockers are excreted partly through the kidney, and the dose is typically started at half of the usual dose given. Aluminum- and magnesium-containing antacids should not be used for patients receiving dialysis treatment as there is a risk that aluminum or magnesium levels may become toxic.

Pancreatitis

Acute pancreatitis is not commonly seen in patients on dialysis; however, it can occur in 2%-9% of patients who have had a kidney transplant. Because amylase levels can be elevated in dialysis patients, additional means of diagnosis, such as pain in the left upper quadrant and elevated lipase levels are typically used. Treatment for acute pancreatitis in patients with CKD does not differ from those patients without CKD. Pain control, hydration, and close monitoring of vital signs are part of the care for acute pancreatitis. Patients should not consume any food or fluid by mouth, and nasogastric suction may be indicated in the case of severe nausea or vomiting. Nutrition is restarted once the pain has lessened. Diet, which should be low in fat and protein at first, can gradually advance over a few days, while monitoring the patient for pain and changes in serum amylase and lipase.

Angiodysplasia

Angiodysplasia occurs when lesions are formed in the GI tract as a result of a small vascular malformation. It usually occurs in the right colon and cecum. Diagnosis is made through endoscopy or angiography. For patients with end stage renal disease, angiodysplasia can cause both acute and chronic blood loss especially in patients over age 50. Because platelet dysfunction must be corrected in these patients and for those on dialysis, the amount of heparin used is reduced. Many of the lesions will stop bleeding without additional treatment; however, some lesions may need to be cauterized through a colonoscopy. Angiography may also be used to help with clotting. Occasionally, surgery is required for a right colectomy. Patients who receive dialysis may have a higher risk of ischemic bowel disease because of the fragile vasculature in the GI tract. Many patients also have atherosclerosis, which may also increase risk. Hypotension that may be experienced during or around the hemodialysis session will also contribute to overall risk.

Adynamic Bone Disease and Osteomalacia

Adynamic bone disease is a reduction in the number of osteoclasts or osteoblasts, or a reduced rate of bone formation. The symptoms may include hypercalcemia, soft tissue calcifications, and bone pain as the disease advances. Fractures are possible. The exact mechanism for adynamic bone disease is not known, but is likely related in part to persistent hypoparathyroidism. There are certain people who are more likely to develop this disease, such as elderly individuals, Caucasians, females, individuals with diabetes, and those receiving peritoneal dialysis. Osteomalacia is similar to adynamic bone disease, but is characterized by decreased bone mineralization. Bones are very soft and brittle. It is generally due to Vitamin D deficiency. Symptoms include pain in the limbs and progressive weakness.

Bone Disease in Individuals Receiving Dialysis

Hyperparathyroidism is usually the primary cause of bone disease. This typically develops in patients when the glomerular filtration rate drops below 70 mL per minute. Hyperparathyroidism can occur because of hypocalcemia or decreased calcitriol levels as a result of impaired hydroxylation of 25-hydroxyvitamin D in the kidney. Calcitriol acts to prevent the synthesis of parathyroid hormone, but because calcitriol receptors are reduced in uremia, the feedback mechanism is impaired. Other possible causes of bone disease include advanced age, women who are postmenopausal, or vitamin D deficiency. Certain medications such as anticonvulsants may interfere with vitamin D absorption. Malignancy or metastasis to the bones, as well as being immobile for a long period of time, may increase the risk for bone disease.

Renal Osteodystrophy in Children

Renal osteodystrophy refers to changes in the skeleton as a result of chronic renal failure. It is a condition more serious in children because their bones are not fully formed and they are actively growing. It may be seen in children receiving continuous ambulatory peritoneal dialysis (CAPD). In order to prevent or treat renal osteodystrophy, close monitoring of serum calcium, phosphorus, bicarbonate, alkaline phosphatase, and parathyroid hormone levels is imperative. The presence of hyperparathyroidism should be promptly treated with vitamin D as calcitriol. Phosphate binders should be prescribed for elevated serum levels of phosphorus as well as a restriction of dietary phosphorus. A phosphorus-restricted diet is sometimes more difficult to achieve in children receiving CAPD because protein is usually not restricted, and protein contributes to the overall phosphorus intake. Exercise may also be beneficial to help strengthen bones.

Bone Disease in Children

Bone disease may present in children as hypocalcemia, hyperphosphatemia, impaired vitamin D metabolism, and a secondary hyperparathyroidism. Vitamin D deficiency causes skeletal deformities and rickets. Children may experience bone pain and fractures, which may lead to continued muscle weakness and a change in the way the child walks. This may progress to a waddling type movement as an attempt by the child to minimize the pain he or she feels with walking. Linear growth failure is possible. There may also be delayed skeletal maturation. Consideration as to genetic height potential must be given; however, this linear growth failure may be addressed by providing growth hormone as early as possible. There may also be soft tissue calcification in the organs, such as the lungs, kidneys, or heart, and may also affect blood vessels, coronary arteries, and heart valves.

PTH

Intact parathyroid hormone (iPTH) should be within 150-300 pg/mL, and a new assay called biointact parathyroid hormone (biPTH) should be within 80-160 pg/mL. If PTH is chronically low, adynamic bone disease may develop. The hemodialysis solution should not contain more than 2.5 mEq/L of calcium (1.25 mM). Using a dialysis solution containing between 1.0-2.0 mEq/L of calcium (0.5-1.0 mM) for up to 6 months may be sufficient to stimulate secretion of PTH because of persistent intradialytic hypocalcemia. For patients receiving peritoneal dialysis who already have adynamic bone disease, a dialysis solution of 2.0 mEq/L of calcium (1.0 mM) should improve bone mineralization and increase secretion of PTH, thus improving serum levels of PTH. In addition to calcium being maintained in a low normal range, serum phosphorus should also be kept in a normal range to stimulate PTH secretion. Providing the active form of vitamin D is contraindicated as this will contribute further to hypoparathyroidism.

Hyperparathyroidism

The calcium content of the dialysis solution for patients with hyperparathyroidism should be 2.0-2.5 mEq/L (1.0-1.25 mM). A lower calcium solution may be used to treat hypercalcemia; however, hypocalcemia between dialysis treatments will stimulate secretion of parathyroid hormone (PTH) and further complicate matters. Serum calcium should be kept between 8.4-10.2 mg/dL (2.1-2.6 mmol/L) and serum phosphorus should be kept between 3.5-5.5 mg/dL (1.1-1.8 mmol/L). Although hypercalcemia will lower PTH secretion, it will contribute to soft tissue calcification and vascular complications. Elevated serum phosphorus levels will stimulate PTH secretion; therefore, keeping serum phosphorus in balance will help to lower PTH level. Providing vitamin D or vitamin D analogs will help lower PTH levels. The doses of vitamin D or vitamin D analogs should be reevaluated monthly based on PTH levels. Once stable, doses should be reassessed every 3 months.

Parathyroidectomy

If measures to control hyperparathyroidism are not successful, surgical removal of the parathyroid gland may be indicated. This is more likely in patients who are female, without diabetes, younger in age, receiving peritoneal dialysis, or receiving dialysis for a longer period of time. The major indications include severe hyperparathyroidism coupled with progression of bone disease as evidenced by continued skeletal pain and fractures even with intensive medical management. Other major indications include severe hyperparathyroidism coupled with the presence of persistent hypercalcemia, severe itching (pruritus) that cannot be resolved, or unsuccessful attempts at controlling hyperphosphatemia with the development of severe soft tissue calcification. Other indications are the presence of skin necrosis (calciphylaxis) or the presence of severe arthritis in addition to hyperparathyroidism. Contraindications to this are patients who have aluminum overload.

Use of Herbs

The use of herbal and other dietary supplements has significantly increased in recent years. These products can include amino acids, vitamins, minerals, enzymes, and other types of products. In 1994, the Dietary Supplement Health and Education Act was passed. This Act, intended to help with safety, definition of products, health claims, labeling, and proper manufacturing processes, established two government bodies to help oversee this process. There is no regulation by the Food and Drug Administration, however, and this can be cause for concern in many people. This means there are no set standards for safety, ingredients, quality control, or proof of efficacy. This can lead to adverse effects especially for people with CKD or kidney transplant. For example, products such as ginseng are supposed to improve immune function, and this would not be a good choice for a patient receiving immunosuppressive drugs. The use of dietary supplements is discouraged in patients with CKD or in those who have had kidney transplants. Patients should discuss the use of any of these products with their physician.

Grapefruit Juice and Grapefruit Products

The use of grapefruit juice or other grapefruit products has been shown to have adverse effects on the absorption of certain drugs. The rationale is that grapefruit is metabolized by the same enzyme that also breaks down many medications. This can lead to a buildup of the medication in the blood stream to dangerous levels. Other fruits to avoid would include tangelos and any product that contains grapefruit bioflavonoids. The main drugs that would be implicated for patients following kidney transplant would be cyclosporine, tacrolimus, and sirolimus. Other medications that may have an interaction would include lipid-lowering medications such as simvastin, lovastatin, and atorvastatin. Certain calcium channel blockers such as Feldodipine and Nifedipine are also affected. It does not take much grapefruit juice to cause a problem and the effects can last as long as 24 hours.

Assessment of Dialysis Therapy

Hemodialysis

Prescription for Hemodialysis

The two main components are the dialyzer clearance (K) and the length of the dialysis session (t). These are determined in part by:

- Blood flow rate - standard flow rate is 500 mL/minute
- Dialyzer membrane, ultra filtration coefficient (Kuf), and dialyzer urea clearance (KOA)
- Dialysis solution flow rate
- Adjusting K x t for the size of the patient (V). The equation = Kt/V

Other components include:

- Type of access
- Dialysis solution temperature
- Dialysis solution - can consist of bicarbonate, sodium, potassium, calcium, magnesium, dextrose, phosphate
- Fluid removal orders
- Anticoagulation orders
- Standing orders for dealing with any complications such as cramping, hypotension, nausea, or chest pain

Fluid Removal Orders

One component of determining fluid removal orders is judging what the patient's dry weight should be. This is determined post-dialysis when all excess fluid has been taken off through the dialysis process. It is important to accurately set a dry weight as closely as possible, because a weight that is too low may be the cause of hypotension at the end of a hemodialysis session. If the weight is too high, the patient is at risk for complications of fluid overload such as pulmonary edema. There is no real scientific method to determining the weight, but it is important to reevaluate the dry weight every 2 weeks to make sure it is still appropriate. The ultrafiltration rate should encompass any fluids taken during the session and should include 200 mL that the patient will receive at the end of the session with the blood return procedure. The fluid removal rate remains constant during the session. The sodium level of the solution also affects the osmotic load of the blood volume during removal.

Hemodialysis Session

A pre-dialysis weight should be taken, and this value should be compared to the patient's estimated dry weight and the last available pre-dialysis weight. This helps to determine if the patient is complying with the fluid and sodium restrictions at home. The goal is less than 1 kg gain per day between dialysis sessions. The patient's blood pressure is closely monitored. Blood pressure can rise during dialysis and patients are usually told not to take their blood pressure medicine on hemodialysis days to prevent a drop in blood pressure. Temperature is also monitored. If an abnormal temperature is noted before the hemodialysis session commences, this should be checked out carefully. The access site should be checked for any issues. Blood pressure and pulse are monitored every 30 to 60 minutes during the session.

Nausea and Vomiting During Hemodialysis

The development of nausea and vomiting is a possibility in patients undergoing hemodialysis treatments. There are a few possible reasons for this, but the main reason is usually the presence of hypotension. Nausea and vomiting may also be due to the development of disequilibrium syndrome, although this is much less commonly seen. In patients with diabetes, the presence of gastroparesis may be the reason for nausea and vomiting, and the symptoms of gastroparesis are often more pronounced during hemodialysis. Dialysis solution that is contaminated or nor formulated properly may be another causative factor. In terms of management, the underlying cause of the nausea and vomiting must be addressed. Medications such as antiemetics or antinausea agents can be prescribed. Some patients also benefit from a small dose of metoclopramide before dialysis begins.

Possible Pathophysiology of Bone Disease in Individuals Receiving Dialysis

Hyperparathyroidism is usually the primary cause of bone disease. This typically develops in patients when the glomerular filtration rate drops below 70 mL per minute. Hyperparathyroidism can occur because of hypocalcemia or decreased calcitriol levels as a result of impaired hydroxylation of 25-hydroxyvitamin D in the kidney. Calcitriol acts to prevent the synthesis of parathyroid hormone, but because calcitriol receptors are reduced in uremia, the feedback mechanism is impaired. Other possible causes of bone disease include advanced age, women who are postmenopausal, or vitamin D deficiency. Certain medications such as anticonvulsants may interfere with vitamin D absorption. Malignancy or metastasis to the bones, as well as being immobile for a long period of time, may increase the risk for bone disease.

Factors That Adversely Affect Immune Function in CKD Receiving Dialysis

There are many factors that influence immune function in individuals with CKD receiving dialysis. These include:

- Increased frequency and severity of bacterial infections- this may be related to frequent access through skin and other mucosal barriers increasing the chance for contamination. Dialysis patients are not usually immunocompromised; however, the infection tends to worsen more rapidly than in the general population.
- Issues with temperature control- many patients receiving hemodialysis have a reduced body temperature at baseline.

- Access site infections- this can be due to contaminated solutions or machines, or from inadequate hygiene.
- Urinary tract infections- dialysis patients tend to have higher rates of urinary tract infection (UTI).
- Pneumonia- rates are higher in dialysis patients, especially those in a hospital setting.
- Vital infections- hepatitis C tends to be higher in dialysis patients than in the general population. Other viral infections include cytomegalovirus, influenza, and HIV.

URR

The Urea reduction ratio (URR) is a measure of how effective hemodialysis is for a patient. It is calculated by subtracting post-dialysis blood urea nitrogen (BUN) from the pre-dialysis BUN. The URR is then provided as a percentage by dividing the difference by the pre-dialysis BUN. The URR should be calculated monthly, and a target percentage is to have the majority of URR greater than 65%. The Kt/V is considered more accurate than URR because it takes into account fluid removal in addition to urea. The Kt/V is also calculated monthly with a target minimum value of 1.2 for most sessions. Both values are assessed and evaluated. Studies have demonstrated that patients receiving dialysis who do not consistently have URR levels greater than 65% and Kt/V values of 1.2 or more have more health issues and also have a greater risk of mortality. These guidelines apply to both children and adults who receive hemodialysis 3 times per week.

URR and Kt/V Values Below Target

If the Kt/V and the URR are consistently below target, the nephrologists will need to reevaluate the treatment plan. The Kt/V can sometimes be improved by increasing the session length. The patient should always be encouraged to complete the entire session. It may also be improved by improving the blood flow, although this is often difficult to accomplish due to access issues. A big dialyzer can sometimes be used to improve clearance, and occasionally 2 dialyzers are used to improve clearance. Increasing the flow rate is another option for improving clearance. A typical flow rate for adults is 350 mL/minute and an increase greater than 500 mL/minute. An increase up to 800 mL/minute is a possibility for some patients.

Important Terms

Blood flow rate: Blood flow rate measures how fast the blood is being pumped through the dialyzer membrane. A higher flow rate will remove more urea.

Urea clearance: Dialyzer urea clearance, also known as KOA, measures the ability of the dialyzer to effectively remove urea via the membrane pores. This number is influenced by the size of the membrane and the number of pores as well as the size of the pores. A larger dialyzer will increase KOA.

Dialysate flow rate: Dialysate flow rate measures how fast the dialysate is pumped through the dialyzer. A higher dialysate flow rate will removed more urea.

Heparinization: Heparinization is the addition of heparin, which keeps the blood from clotting and keeps the blood flowing smoothly through the membrane. An appropriate heparin dose will help to remove more urea.

Vascular access: Vascular access is how hemodialysis occurs. An arteriovenous (AV) fistula is the best type of vascular access. The fistula needs to be working well for dialysis to be effective.

Dry Weight or Target Weight for Children

As with the adult population, there is no real scientific method for determining a child's dry or target weight. It is imperative that practitioners experienced in pediatrics, including a pediatric dietitian, be involved in the care of children. Continued reassessment of the target weight needs to occur for growth reasons. Children have a higher total body water content than adults. Body composition changes rapidly especially in infants and adolescents. This is especially important if the child is receiving growth hormone therapy. Another factor to keep in mind is that dietary intake of food and fluid for a child can vary widely from day to day. An accurate target weight will help to minimize issues with hypotension during sessions. It will also ensure that growth is occurring normally and if not, growth issues are being addressed in a timely manner.

Peritoneal Dialysis

Prescription for PD

The components of a peritoneal dialysis (PD) prescription are as follows:

- Volume of dialysis solution - For adults, the "bags" are typically are packaged in volumes of 1.5 liters advancing in increments of 500 mL up to 3-liter bags.
- Dextrose concentration of the dialysate - Dextrose in the form of glucose monohydrate is used to act as the osmotic agent. Dextrose concentration includes: 1.5%, 2.5%, 4.25%.
- Electrolyte concentration of the dialysate - Composition of dialysate is fairly consistent between manufacturers. Solutions typically contain sodium, calcium, magnesium, lactated ringers, or bicarbonate. Potassium can be added if needed.
- Additives to dialysate - This can include heparin, insulin, and antibiotics.
- Temperature of solution
- Length of session
- Exchange time - This includes inflow time, dwell time and outflow time.
- Careful tracking of intake and output and monitoring of clearance by checking blood urea nitrogen (BUN) and other lab data. Orders on when to contact physician for complications

Dextrose Concentration for PD

A 1.5% dextrose concentration is the typical solution used for most patients receiving PD. This concentration allows removal of 50-150 mL of fluid an hour using 2- liter exchanges with 60-minute exchange time. More volume will be removed than is instilled into the patient. Between 1.2 and 3.6 liters of fluid can be removed over the course of a day. A higher dextrose concentration will allow more fluid to be removed. For example, a 2-liter exchange with a 60-minute dwell time can remove 300-400 mL per hour, or approximately 7-9 liters per day. This would be used in situations such as congestive heart failure where immediate removal of fluid is imperative. Sometimes a combination of dextrose concentrations is used to achieve optimal fluid removal. Once the patient has achieved a normal fluid balance, a change to 1.5% concentration is desired.

CAPD

Peritoneal dialysis (PD) is available in several different forms, and CAPD is the most commonly used form. This form of PD requires multiple sessions throughout the day that take up to 40 minutes per session and leaves the dialysate dwelling for various amounts of time. This type of PD is more affordable, does not require being hooked up to machinery for long periods of time (i.e. 3-4 hours per session), and can easily control renal disease. It does require a sterile environment, which is a consideration for travel, work, or school. Overall, though, with careful planning, it does allow more flexibility for those patients who work or go to school. CAPD involves a less restrictive diet than hemodialysis. CAPD can induce better control of blood pressure and possibly a reduction in the decline of residual urine output. A disadvantage of CAPD includes potential for weight gain due to metabolism of dextrose.

Complications of PD

Possible acute complications of PD may include:

- Abdominal distension - This may be a result of accumulation of drainage in the peritoneum due to inadequate drainage.
- Peritonitis - 12% of acute PD patients will develop this.
- Hypotension- This can be due to removal of too much fluid leading to hypovolemia. Immediate correction is required. This usually involves giving IV 0.9% normal saline solution followed by readjustment of PD orders.
- Hypernatremia - This can be caused by too frequent exchanges.
- Hyperglycemia - This can occur in patients who have pre-diabetes or preexisting diabetes and is due to the high dextrose concentration. Close monitoring of blood glucose levels is advised. Addition of insulin to the dialysate may be needed.
- Low serum albumin – This can occur because of the increased protein losses.

CCPD and NIPD

A second type of PD is automated PD (APD), which involves a combination of continuous cycling PD (CCPD) and nocturnal intermittent PD (NIPD). CCPD involves leaving the PD solution dwelling throughout the day without any exchanges. Then at bedtime, the patient connects to a cycler that drains and refills multiple times during the night, leaving the last cycle to dwell throughout the day. CCPD can cause discomfort during the day related to the long abdominal dwell time. For NIPD, the final nocturnal dwell is drained in the morning, and the patient does not perform any exchanges during the day. This has a lower clearance rate but is often used for those who have better residual kidney function. There are also other combinations of CCPD and NIPD that are designed to better fit into a patient's life and increase compliance with therapy.

Adequacy of PD

The general target for measuring the adequacy of PD is Kt/V. Previously set at 2.0, the target level has recently been lowered to 1.7 because higher levels have not been shown to improve outcomes. The Kt/V target value is higher than that of hemodialysis because PD is overall more efficient at clearing urea than hemodialysis. Another measure of adequacy is the creatinine clearance (CrCl). This peritoneal CrCl is calculated by assessing the creatinine content of 24 hours' worth of dialysate effluent. This number is then divided by serum creatinine. The renal CrCl averages the creatinine clearance with the urea clearance. The equation is as follows:

renal CrCl = 0.5 [24-hour urine creatinine content/serum creatinine + 24-hour urine urea nitrogen content/ serum urea nitrogen]

Clearance

There are a number of factors that may impact clearance for patients receiving PD. These may include factors related to the prescription such as inadequate dwell volume, insufficient number of exchanges, or utilization of the wrong dextrose concentration for the dialysate. This can be addressed by increasing the number of daily exchanges, increasing the dwell volume, or increasing the dextrose concentration of the dialysate. For patients who receive automatic PD, it may be due to insufficient number of daytime dwells. It can also be addressed by increasing the length of time or the dwell time on the cycler. This can be addressed by altering the schedule of day dwells or increasing the length of time spent on the cycler at night. Factors unrelated to the PD prescription include body size and residual kidney function. Body size affects clearance in that it is more difficult to attain improved clearance targets. Also, clearance is affected if weight is based on desirable instead of actual body weight. Residual renal function can be as high as 50%, and this will impact clearance.

Compliance of Patient

The success of PD largely relies on the compliance of the patient to the PD routine. Possible signs of noncompliance include symptoms of uremia, elevated blood urea nitrogen (BUN) and/or potassium, or an increase in total creatinine excretion compared to the baseline number. It should be noted that an increase in the amount of lean body mass can affect creatinine excretion and should be considered.

Examples of ways that PD patients are noncompliant include shortening the amount of time on the cycler, omitting CAPD exchanges, shortening the amount of dwell time, allowing insufficient time between exchanges, or omitting day dwells for patients receiving automatic PD. Other factors that may affect the success of PD are the patient's overall health status and ability to perform the PD routine, the size of the patient, residual urine output, and poor nutritional status. The functionality of the catheter is also important in PD success.

PET AND PTR

Peritoneal equilibration test PET is defined as the test that measures how well the patient's peritoneal membrane functions. It measures the solute clearance, amount of glucose absorbed, amount of protein lost, and ultrafiltration. The PET is done within the first 1-2 months of treatment and will define the membrane function as low, low average, high, and high average. This is called the peritoneal transport rate (PTR), which helps the physician to tailor the PD prescription for the type of membrane function, thus achieving the best possible clinical outcome.

Most PD patients will have a PTR equal to high average or low average. Those who have a high PTR have a higher risk for morbidity and mortality, and overall poor outcome. High PTR will also have a higher rate of protein losses thus a lower serum albumin level. High PTR typically means the transporters are able to dialyze but not ultrafiltrate. Conversely, low PTR will ultrafiltrate well but are not able to adequately dialyze; thus, these patients will have lower rates of protein losses. Low average or high average is the overall goal.

Provision of Patient Education

Effective RD

A dietitian who is specially trained in treating patients with chronic kidney disease is well versed in how nutrition affects outcomes. The renal dietitian (RD) should be able to help to identify a patient's goal and to facilitate this goal through education. The patient should not be told what he or she needs to do; rather, the patient should be educated on how diet and nutrition will affect outcome. The RD needs to be able to effectively assess the ability to learn, issues with compliance, and any neurological impairments that may affect learning, such as dementia or aging. The RD needs to evaluate issues such as finances, access to food, social supports, state of mind such as the presence of depression, and any cultural issues, and incorporate these into the plan of care. RDs should be able to provide motivation and effective communication to help a patient incorporate the life changes they need to make to manage their disease.

Effective Education

The RD needs to determine how the patient best learns. Many people are visual learners, others are auditory, and still others are hands-on. The RD should be able to provide effective education based on the patient's learning style. For visual learners, food models can be helpful to demonstrate portion sizes and meal composition. Also, written materials that include colorful images are helpful, as are videos. For those who are auditory learners, conversations with the patient or the use of CDs can help with the education process. For patients who prefer hands-on learning, food models or pictures are useful, as are workbooks, quizzes, or other written activities. Teaching sessions should be succinct and deal with one or two changes at a time. A fifth-grade reading level is recommended for communication. Time for feedback or questions should be allotted. Role-playing and problem solving together with the patient are also helpful. Continued education can be accomplished by using bulletin boards, newsletters, cooking demonstrations, or guest presentations.

Educational Components for CKD and Dyslipidemia

Therapeutic Lifestyle Changes (TLC) should be incorporated for patients with CKD and dyslipidemia. TLC is derived from the ATP III of the National Cholesterol Education Program. The main points to educate the patient on include:

- Reduction of saturated fat and cholesterol (saturated fat less than 7%, polyunsaturated fat up to 10%, and monounsaturated fat up to 20% of total calories)
- Limiting carbohydrates to 50%-60% of total calories
- Increasing fiber to 20-30 grams per day and consider the addition of plant sterols to diet
- Achieving and maintaining appropriate weight

- Increasing daily activity to a moderate level (for example, a 10,000-step-per-day goal as part of regular activity) and planning physical activity such as 30-minute sessions 3-4 times per week of swimming, walking, etc.
- Limiting alcohol intake and quitting smoking

TLC Dietary Components

The American Heart Association (AHA) no longer uses the terms Step I and II when describing heart healthy diets. These terms were replaced in 2001 with the TLC diet. The general recommendations for this diet are as follows:

- Total fat intake should comprise between 25%-35% of total calories
- Total carbohydrate intake should comprise 50%-60% of total calories
- Total protein intake should comprise up to 15% of total calories
- Caloric intake should be sufficient to reach and maintain a desirable body weight
- Saturated fat intake should be limited to less than 7% of total calories with monounsaturated fat providing up to 20% and polyunsaturated fat up to 10%. It is also recommended that trans fats be limited. Cholesterol intake should be less than 200 mg per day
- 10-25 grams of soluble fiber should be included and carbohydrate intake should be mainly complex carbohydrates and fresh fruits and vegetables.
- Weight management and increased physical activity are also important components

Hyperkalemia

The goal for serum potassium is 3.5-5 mmol/L. The symptoms of hyperkalemia include nausea, abnormal pulse rate, or slow heart rate. Other symptoms include tingling in the extremities, fatigue, and weakness. Hyperkalemia can be very dangerous because it can lead to cardiac arrest or cardiac arrhythmias. It can also adversely affect nerve and muscle control. Hyperkalemia can be treated with a dietary restriction of 2000 mg of potassium or less per day. The diet should include a variety of foods, but high-potassium foods containing greater than 200 mg per serving should be limited. A list of high-potassium foods should be reviewed with the patient as well as appropriate substitutions that would be lower in potassium. Foods that contain significant amounts of potassium include bananas, potatoes, oranges, melon, tomatoes, dairy products, and protein sources. Salt substitutes should be avoided. Portion control is essential. If a high-potassium food is desired, the patient should be instructed on how potassium can be leached out or the food incorporated into the diet.

Hyperphosphatemia

The goal for serum phosphorus is 3.5-5.5 mg/dL. Hyperphosphatemia does not usually have symptoms that the patient can recognize but has significant consequences. These include weakened bones or the development of calcium deposits in blood vessels, eyes, or the heart, which can be painful and dangerous. Dialysis can control phosphorus somewhat, but it is imperative for the patient to adhere to the prescribed low-phosphorus diet and/or phosphate binders. A list of high-phosphorus foods should be reviewed with the patient. Some high-phosphorus foods include dairy products, dried beans, bran, nuts, chocolate, cola drinks, and beer. It is important for the patient to receive instruction on making appropriate substitutions such as nondairy creamer for milk and to receive a list of low-phosphorus foods that may be included in the diet.

Excessive Sodium and Fluid Intake

In CKD, excess sodium and fluid build up in the body because the kidneys are not able to adequately excrete the excess. This can lead to edema, swollen ankles, high blood pressure, or congestive heart failure. The normal range for serum sodium is 135-145 mEq/L. Most patients with CKD would need to follow a sodium restricted diet. This would include patients with acute renal failure, patients in the later stages of CKD, and those on hemodialysis. Patients receiving peritoneal dialysis do not usually require a strict low sodium diet or fluid restriction. The restriction for sodium can range from 1000-4000 mg per day. Fluid is usually restricted for most patients with CKD with or without dialysis. The amount of fluid allotted during a day is dependent upon intake and output. This is usually calculated by adding 1000 mL to the amount of urine output. For those on hemodialysis, fluid intake is based on the amount of weight gain between dialysis treatments.

Low Sodium Diet

The main points to cover when educating a patient on a low sodium diet include:

- Avoiding use of the salt shaker and caution with use of salt substitutes
- Using herbs to flavor foods
- Reading labels, including explaining commonly used terms on the label such as very low sodium or sodium free. Serving sizes should be reviewed as well as key words to identify sodium-containing ingredients.
- Avoiding processed foods, especially cured meats, such as bacon or ham, certain luncheon meats, canned soups, and vegetables
- Avoiding frozen dinners and dry noodle or rice mixes, such as Rice-A-Roni or Ramen noodles
- Avoiding high sodium condiments, such as barbeque sauce, and high sodium snack foods
- Learning how to order at a restaurant
- Learning about appropriate substitutions

Fluid Restriction

A fluid restriction is essential to managing chronic kidney disease (CKD). Reinforcement of the sodium restriction is important, as too much sodium intake will increase thirst. If the patient receives hemodialysis, the patient should be educated on appropriate weight gain between hemodialysis treatments. Patients also need to recognize factors that may increase fluid requirements, such as fever, vomiting, or excessive sweating. However, any increases in fluid intake should be reviewed first with the physician. The patient should be instructed on signs of fluid overload such as difficulty breathing, excessive ankle swelling, a sharp increase in weight, or a rise in blood pressure above baseline. Daily recording of weight is important. Types of fluid should be defined as any food that is liquid at room temperature. The patient needs to learn how to accurately measure and assess fluid intake and should be instructed on how to spread the fluid allotment out over the course of a day. Tips for dealing with thirst should be reviewed such as eating cold sliced fruits, or using sour candies or artificial saliva.

Protein Intake

The patient needs to understand his or her protein allowance and the rationale for this. For example, a patient with CKD not yet on dialysis may require a protein restriction to less than 1 gram per kg. Conversely, a patient on hemodialysis may require up to 1.5 grams per kg of protein per day. The effects of insufficient protein intake and its association with mortality should be reviewed with the patient, including serum albumin level. Because at least 50% of the protein source should be of high biological value (HBV), the patient needs to identify what foods contain HBV protein. This would include meat, fish, poultry, eggs, and dairy. Being able to incorporate these types of protein is important in relation to other restrictions such as phosphorus. Advice on how to assess portion size is important, such as 3 ounces of meat is equal to the size of a deck of cards.

Low Protein Diet

For those on a low protein diet, tips on stretching protein should be provided, such as thinly slicing meats or adding additional rice or pasta to be more filling. Tips for preparing satisfying main dishes should be reviewed, such as making vegetables and grains the focus of the meal or modifying a casserole to be lower in protein. Substituting nondairy creamer for milk in cream soups will help to reduce protein. Education on recipe modification is important as well. The use of special low protein foods can be discussed if the patient requires these. Maintaining adequate calorie intake is important to prevent weight loss and maintain nutritional status. Adding calories to foods without adding protein should also be reviewed, such as adding certain fats.

Anemia

The symptoms of anemia should be reviewed with the patient including tiredness or listlessness, dizziness, washed-out skin coloring, or inability to think clearly. The plan for treatment should be reviewed including the use of Epogen or Procrit, and the goal for the individual's hemoglobin level should be identified. Increasing iron in the diet is also important as well as making sure enough vitamin B12 and folic acid is consumed. The best source of iron is heme iron, and this can be found in red meats, dark poultry, and certain types of seafood. Other good sources of iron include iron-fortified cereal, blackstrap molasses, beans, and lentils. It is important to work with a registered dietitian to incorporate these foods into the diet in relation to other restrictions. An iron supplement or intravenous iron is often prescribed.

Bone Health

First, the patient needs a basic understanding of the role of the kidney in maintaining calcium and phosphorus balance, vitamin D metabolism, and parathyroid hormone (PTH). Second, the patient needs an understanding of the consequences of renal osteodystrophy, such as weakened bones and calcification of the heart, arteries, and valves as well as soft tissues. Third, it is important for the patient to understand the significance of laboratory data such as PTH, serum calcium, phosphorus, and bone density tests. Next, the patient needs to be educated on treatment options for preventing or controlling renal osteodystrophy. This would include the use of medications such as phosphate binders, vitamin D analogs, calcimimetic agents, and appropriate dietary interventions. A registered dietitian experienced in this area can make a major impact on the patient's comprehension and compliance.

Exercise

Exercise is important to the general population but is especially important to those with CKD. Exercise can positively affect daily life by increasing a person's energy and stamina. Moderate levels of physical activity will help with blood pressure and weight control. This is especially significant early in the disease process as weight and blood pressure may be more difficult to control as the disease progresses. Physical activity helps with controlling blood glucose for those with pre-diabetes or diabetes. Exercise also helps in the treatment of hyperlipidemia, which is important for delaying further complications. Treating bone disease with moderate physical activity helps to strengthen the bones. It is important for children with CKD to get into the habit of exercising early to help to prevent complications. Regular exercise can help to maintain muscle mass. A goal for most patients is 20-30 minutes of moderate exercise 3-4 times per week at a minimum coupled with good choices for daily lifestyle activities, such as taking the stairs instead of elevator.

Intensity of Exercise for CKD Patients

A minimum of 30 minutes of moderate exercise 3-4 times per week is a good goal, and this can be gradually achieved based on the individual's endurance. It is best to alternate days if possible. The patient should be directed to push him or herself to a point where they have raised their heart rate but can still maintain a conversation without needing to stop to breathe. Exercising in cooler temperatures such as early morning or evening is recommended. Exercising at least an hour after eating a meal is also recommended, as is not exercising too close to bedtime. Patients should be advised against exercising if a fever is present, if the weather is very hot and humid, if there is a significant change in the dialysis or medication schedule, or if exercise is making bone or joint issues worse.

Care Plan for Parent or Caretaker

There are many issues that need to be addressed with the parents of a child with CKD. These include:

- Education about the disease and treatment
- Diet and growth
- Medication
- Dealing with the effects of CKD on the child and family unit and incorporating the disease into the family's routine
- Finding additional support

The nutrition care plan will continually evolve based on the child's age, stage of development, growth, favorite foods, stage of renal disease and type of treatment being used, laboratory data, medication use, and social situation. The care plan needs to be individualized and modified as needed to meet the child's changing requirements.

Noncompliance

Problem Solving Techniques and Addressing Barriers

Problem solving techniques and addressing barriers are two strategies that can be employed to help address noncompliance in patients with CKD. Problem solving involves the identification of problem areas that the patient may have difficulty dealing with. The problem areas are discussed in depth and possible solutions or strategies to deal with the situations are discussed in depth. The use of relapse prevention techniques is also important. Situations that are deemed high risk, such as a certain type of social function, are identified well in advance and the patient becomes better equipped to deal with the scenario. Addressing barriers is also imperative to overall compliance. Because the regimen for patients with CKD can be very complicated, assistance is essential to make the regimen more adaptable and to provide support to the patient. The barriers should be identified by the patient and may involve such issues as complying with a medication schedule, requiring assistance with purchasing food, or dealing with the side effects of medications.

Techniques to Encourage Dietary Compliance

Goal setting is one technique that can be used to encourage compliance. The registered dietitian and the patient can set small goals to help achieve change, such as increasing protein intake by 10 grams over the next week. Another technique is verbal persuasion. This can help by exploring a patient's health care concerns, beliefs, and practices, then addressing these issues and attempting to convince or persuade the patient to see the benefits of change. A review of the consequences that may occur if the patient does or does not follow the restrictions is essential. The patient can also be persuaded or convinced that today is a new day, and it can be time to move forward. Again, small but measurable goals and steps are helpful in assisting the patient. Helping the patient achieve independent self-management is a useful strategy as well. The patient can be encouraged to keep logs of food intake or exercise in order to track progress.

Dealing with Children

The primary caretaker of the child needs to be actively and intensely involved in the educational process. A good and working rapport needs to be established by the registered dietitian in order to be successful. It is important for the child to be actively involved in the education process when possible based on age and development, as chronic kidney disease (CKD) is a lifelong situation. Honesty, open communication, and being well prepared for procedures, etc., are extremely helpful for a child. The child should gradually be able to assume some degree of control over the care and treatment. This will help the child to develop self-esteem and feel empowered. Guidance on making healthful choices is another point to address. Helping the child to deal with issues of feeling different from everyone else is also important. Providing good role models of famous people such as actors or athletes with CKD is often a useful strategy. Maintaining a positive attitude and a sense of humor is also important.

Compliance in Children and Adolescents

Compliance in children and adolescents is extremely important as non-compliance can adversely affect growth and development, overall health, and functioning. Prevention of long-term consequences is important as well. When diet restrictions need to be added to a child's diet, it is usually done in a generalized way. For example, if a child requires a potassium restriction, it is added as "low potassium" rather than a specified amount of restriction. The child and caretakers are then educated on what foods to avoid. In this example, the child would be instructed to avoid bananas, potatoes, chocolate, orange juice, and melon. If the child continues to have high serum potassium levels, a diet recall can assess whether additional foods need to be avoided.

Education

Children

The age of the child determines whom the registered dietitian educates. For an infant, the focus is with the primary caretaker or parent who is responsible for selecting the foods the infant will consume. The same applies for a toddler, although there needs to be more flexibility as the toddler is able to exert more independence about what he or she will consume. For a school age child, both the primary caretaker and the child need to be involved, as there are many circumstances in which a parent will not be present and the child will be making his or her own food choices. Additionally, teachers and other people who are actively involved in the child's life should be aware of the child's restrictions. For an adolescent, direct education is required in conjunction with the primary caretaker. The adolescent is making the majority of decisions on food choices especially away from the primary caretaker. The adolescent needs to be taking complete responsibility for dietary control with support of the parent or primary caretaker.

Adolescent

Adolescents typically have erratic eating habits. Meals are often skipped or poor substitutions are made for healthy meals. Fast food consumption is higher in this age group and adolescents may eat at fast food places frequently with friends. Beverage selection often tends to be sodas, sports drinks, or other types of sweetened beverages. Intake of milk can often be high. Education needs to be focused on making appropriate selections when away from home and eating with friends. This would include appropriate meal selections at the school cafeteria or fast food restaurant planned in advance so the adolescent is prepared. Recommendations regarding portion sizes should be reinforced. Specific guidance on beverage selection in regard to phosphorus intake is important including alternative drink selections. Safe snack choices should also be provided and reviewed.

Intake or Appetite

It is important to address issues with appetite changes in patients with chronic kidney disease (CKD) as it can lead to weight loss and changes in nutritional status. Advice that may be given includes eating small, more frequent meals and snacks to help increase nutrient intake. Smaller meals are often easier to consume and digest than bigger meals. If meals are missed because of a hemodialysis schedule, the use of nutritional supplements may be indicated. Patients are often too tired to eat after treatment, but skipping meals entirely should not be an option. For those patients with a poor appetite, eating cold foods sometimes helps, as the aroma is often less than with hot foods. If taste changes are present or there is a persistent bad taste in the mouth, the patient should be encouraged to brush frequently including both the teeth and the tongue or to suck on lemon flavored candy before eating to help clear the palate. In some cases, liberalization of the diet may be indicated to try to expand food choices.

Constipation

Constipation is a very possible side effect of many treatments used for patients receiving hemodialysis. The use of phosphate binders can cause constipation. Side effects of other medications, the use of a fluid restriction, and changes in exercise habits can also contribute. Many of the foods that are higher in fiber may also contain significant amounts of potassium and phosphorus. A list should be provided that should include appropriate options for increasing fiber content of the diet without significantly increasing potassium and fiber per gram of dietary fiber. For example, grain products that contain less than 26 mg of phosphorus and less than 33 mg of potassium per gram of fiber include cooked barley, crude corn bran, and spinach egg noodles. Fruits that contain less than 75 mg of potassium per gram of fiber would include pears, apples, strawberries, blueberries, and cranberries. Vegetables that contain less than 100 mg potassium per gram of fiber include cooked green beans, cauliflower, and carrots, or cabbage and collard or turnip greens. The patient should also be educated regarding portion sizes.

Renal Transplant

Pretransplant Period Nutritional Assessment

A complete nutritional assessment should be completed in conjunction with the transplant evaluation. Any nutritional deficiencies should be identified and corrected prior to transplant. Baseline information that should be obtained includes a complete medical history, diet history, weight history, laboratory data, use of nutritional supplements, vitamins, minerals or herbs, and any other information that may affect current or future nutritional status. Additionally, obesity should be addressed. Not only is obesity an overall health risk, it can negatively affect a patient's ability to qualify for a transplant or be placed high enough on the transplant list to make receiving an organ a reality. Pretransplant body mass index (BMI) should ideally be between 22 and 30. Some studies have shown that BMIs higher or lower than this may have a higher risk for death and may have a higher rate of postoperative complications such as loss of graft or increased stay in the ICU or hospital.

Nutritional Requirements in the Acute Post-Transplant Period

Nutritional requirements are generally increased for a period of up to 8 weeks following kidney transplantation. Protein requirements can range form 1.3-2.0 grams per kg due to the increased rate of catabolism. This is caused by the use of corticosteroids and stress from surgery. Calorie requirements are approximately 30-35 kcal/kg or adding a stress factor of 1.3-1.5 to the Harris Benedict equation. Acute hyperglycemia is possible following transplant. Simple carbohydrates may be limited with emphasis on complex carbohydrates. Fat may provide up to 30% of total calories and should consist of more polyunsaturated and monounsaturated fat. In the acute period, sodium may need to be restricted to 2-4 grams per day if the patient is hypertensive or is having issues with fluid retention. Fluid may need to be restricted if these issues are present as well. Potassium should be restricted to less than 4 grams per day if hyperkalemia is present. Vitamins and minerals are required only at the level of the Dietary Reference Intake (DRI).

Nutritional Requirements for an Adult

The nutritional requirements of an adult patient following kidney transplantation are more in line with what is recommended for the general population. Protein requirements are normalized in the range of 0.8-1.0 g/kg using usual weight within ideal body weight range or adjusted weight if the patient is obese. Calories should be calculated to achieve or maintain an ideal body weight. This can be done by adding a stress factor of 1.3 to the Harris Benedict equation. Carbohydrates should consist of mainly complex sources and should contribute no more than 60% of total calories. Fat should be limited to 30% of total calories and saturated fats limited to less than 10% of total calories. Sodium may be restricted if hypertension is present. Vitamins and minerals should be provided at the level of the Dietary Reference Intake (DRI) although calcium may need to be provided at higher levels to help prevent osteoporosis.

Carbohydrate Metabolism

Hyperglycemia is a commonly seen complication following kidney transplantation. The causes may be due to insulin resistance related to the use of corticosteroids. This may be especially true for obese patients or those with a preoperative history of diabetes. Additionally, the use of other immunosuppressive drugs such as cyclosporine or tacrolimus may cause hyperglycemia. Hyperglycemia needs to be addressed. Insulin or oral hypoglycemic agents may be required, and dietary intervention is recommended. Dietary intervention would involve limiting carbohydrate intake to 50%-60% of total calories with emphasis on complex carbohydrates and increasing fiber intake. Calories should be assessed at 30-35 kcal/kg with a goal of achieving a desirable/ideal body weight. Hyperglycemia may gradually resolve in some patients as steroids are weaned, but as many as a third of post transplant patients may continue to have diabetes long term.

Gastrointestinal Issues

Immunosuppression is the main cause of the gastrointestinal issues that may develop post transplant. Immunosuppression increases the risk of acquiring certain types of infections. These may include viral infections such as cytomegalovirus (CMV), which can cause a myriad of issues including diarrhea, gastrointestinal (GI) bleeding, nausea, vomiting, or painful swallowing. It can occur in any part of the GI tract and can even lead to ischemic colitis and perforation if untreated. Herpes simplex virus (HSV) is also possible and can affect any part of the GI tract. It most commonly affects the mouth and esophagus. Bacterial infections can occur, and the most common culprit is *clostridium difficile* colitis. This can cause severe diarrhea and abdominal pain. Fungal infections are also possible and may initially be seen as oral thrush. Gastritis and the development of gastric or peptic ulcers can also occur in the post transplant period, often due to the presence of *Helicobacter pylori*. Lastly, many of the immunosuppressive agents used have GI side effects that may include nausea, vomiting, and diarrhea.

Abnormalities in Serum Potassium

Hyperkalemia can occur post transplantation due to catabolism related to the stress of surgery as well as the use of corticosteroids. Immunosuppressive drugs such as cyclosporine and tacrolimus can also cause hyperkalemia. These drugs may cause a tubular defect in the secretion of potassium or may cause a decrease in the renin-aldosterone system. Poor graft function can also be a cause. A potassium restriction may be implemented. Ensuring that the patient is receiving appropriate levels of calories and protein is important to help reduce catabolism. If the hyperkalemia is not able to be controlled with diet, the use of binding resin such as kayexalate may be used. Potassium-wasting diuretics are sometimes selected to assist with controlling potassium levels.

Calcium Metabolism

The development of metabolic bone disease is a very common complication following kidney transplantation. The degree of bone disease is primarily dependent upon the type and dosages of immunosuppressive drugs used to manage organ rejection. The use of corticosteroids also plays a role. The corticosteroids can inhibit osteoblast function, can increase the excretion of both calcium and phosphorus, and can inhibit the absorption of calcium and phosphorus in the GI tract. Vitamin D metabolism may also be impaired due to corticosteroid use. The patient's history pretransplant is important related to the type and extent of kidney dysfunction and the presence of hyperparathyroid-related bone disease before the transplant. To counteract the effects of corticosteroids, calcium supplementation may be prescribed.

Cardiovascular Disease

Cardiovascular disease is the leading cause of death in patients who have had kidney transplants. The risk factors that lead up to this include obesity, hyperlipidemia, high blood pressure, diabetes, and the presence of a chronic prothrombotic condition. Almost 75% of patients who are post transplant will have elevated lipid levels due primarily to medication use. The medications that adversely affect lipid levels include immunosuppressive agents such as cyclosporine, tacrolimus, sirolimus, and corticosteroids. Certain diuretics and high blood pressure medications will also contribute. Weight gain that can occur following transplant is also a factor. Other contributing causes include age and male gender.

Long Term Management of Cardiovascular Disease

Diet and obesity are two risk factors that can be controlled in a patient with hyperlipidemia and an increased risk of cardiovascular disease. The first step is the implementation or resumption of the therapeutic lifestyle changes. This includes a reduction in dietary fat to 25%-35% of total calories with less than 7% coming from saturated sources. Cholesterol is restricted to less than 200 mg per day. Carbohydrate intake is controlled to no more than 50%-60% of total calories. An increase in total fiber is recommended to 20-30 g per day with a concurrent increase in soluble fiber to 10 g per day. The use of plant stanols have been shown to be beneficial by preventing the absorption of cholesterol by the small intestine. Blood glucose levels should be controlled and an ideal body weight should be achieved and maintained. A desirable body mass index is between 25-28 kg/m^2. Exercise should be increased as approved by the physician.

Weight Gain

There are many potential causes for weight gain following kidney transplantation. This may include a change back to a normal appetite following a period of poor appetite in the pretransplant period. It may be due to the effects of corticosteroid use causing an excessive appetite and uncontrollable intake of food. Corticosteroids may also cause an increase in adipose tissue, and the overall body composition may change. Weight gain may also be the result of stopping dialysis, which may have elevated calorie requirements in the pre-transplant period. Other causes may be lack of physical activity, genetics, age, race or female gender. The implications of obesity in the post transplant period are far reaching. The development of diabetes, hypertension, or cardiovascular disease is possible. Many patients are overweight or obese at the time of transplant, so additional weight gain is even more dangerous.

Utilization of Outcome Management

CQI and PI Programs

A continuous quality improvement (CQI) or performance improvement (PI) program is on ongoing endeavor that continually evaluates outcomes as well as evidence-based research that should be incorporated into the program. The first step is to identify a topic for improvement. A thorough review of evidence-based literature should be conducted. The results of this should then be compared to the current practice in the facility. The primary goal is to improve patient care. The second step is to implement the change in practice. This step involves planning and communication. Any person who would be affected by this change in practice needs to be informed of the events. Any possible barriers should be identified and addressed. The third step is to monitor and evaluate the change in practice. Data should be collected to gauge the effectiveness of the change. Finally, any changes to the original plan should be incorporated. Any additional changes in policy and procedures should be implemented to ensure the change continues.

PD

Research has demonstrated that continuous quality improvement (CQI) or performance improvement (PI) programs will improve the care of patients with stage 5 chronic kidney disease (CKD). For facilities that perform peritoneal dialysis (PD), a careful review should be completed to identify any particular areas with problems. All practitioners should be involved, including physicians, nurses, social workers, dietitians, and anyone else involved in the care of patients receiving PD. Technique failure is one of the key areas that should be addressed. Other areas that can be considered for inclusion in the CQI or PI program include infection rate, peritonitis rate, patient satisfaction, overall quality of life, and issues with catheters. Areas that would have direct nutritional implications include management of anemia, bone status, blood pressure control, and management of lipids. Although the overall care of patients receiving PD will be enhanced, improvements in overall patient outcomes have not been definitively documented.

Protocols for a Dialysis Center

The development of nutrition protocols is an important part of a renal dietitian's job in a dialysis center. Incorporating new research and utilizing an evidence-based approach is paramount to the care of patients with chronic kidney disease (CKD). A great starting point is the National Kidney Foundation. This organization has established a set of core guidelines that can be used by practitioners providing care to patients with kidney disease. There are 12 clinical practice guidelines in the following areas: hemodialysis adequacy, peritoneal dialysis adequacy, vascular access, diabetes and CKD, evaluation, classification and stratification of CKD, anemia management, anemia in CKD, dyslipidemia, hypertension, cardiovascular disease, bone metabolism in both children and adults, and nutrition. Another source of information is the Academy of Nutrition and Dietetics. This organization has already done a lot of the work involved in establishing protocols and can make implementation in a facility much easier. Books, clinical guides, and other published work are available.

Medicare Requirements

MNT

Medical nutrition therapy (MNT) for patients with CKD is one disease entity that is covered by Medicare because it has been documented that nutrition intervention has been beneficial. This has been in place since 2002. MNT services are defined by Congress as "nutritional, diagnostic, therapy, and counseling services furnished by a registered dietitian or nutrition professional...pursuant to a referral by a physician." Requirements have been established that dictate who may provide nutritional care, how often the patient may receive MNT, and eligibility. Medicare also defines renal disease to be chronic renal insufficiency, end stage renal disease to be the medical condition of a beneficiary for 36 months following a kidney transplant when dialysis is not received. Guidelines provide for up to 3 hours for initial MNT for renal disease and up to 2 hours for follow up. Additional hours may be requested based on physician assessment or change in medical condition or treatment plan.

Nutritional Care

Referral of a patient with CKD for medical nutrition therapy (MNT) is very simple. Patients with CKD not receiving dialysis can be covered under Medicare if they qualify and apply for Part B coverage. A physician order is required to receive services and the order must include a diagnosis and diagnosis code for the type of kidney disease the patient has. Recent laboratory data and a list of medications must also be provided. Documentation in the patient's medical record must be completed expressly indicating medical necessity. An appointment can then be arranged with a registered dietitian in a clinic, private practice or at the physician's office. If more hours are required, another referral must be completed.

Medicare Guidelines to Provide MNT Services

Medicare guidelines specify that the MNT be provided by a registered dietitian (RD) or nutrition professional. This person must have a Bachelor's degree and be a registered dietitian. Many have more advanced degrees. The professional has to have completed an accredited program in dietetics or nutrition and maintain professional education requirements. Many also receive national certification by completing the Certified Specialist in Renal (CSR) nutrition exam administered by the Academy of Nutrition and Dietetics. The RD must also be licensed if the state they reside in requires licensure and must have a Medicare number. If state licensure is not available, the Centers for Medicare and Medicaid Services (CMS) will accept status of registration with the Academy of Nutrition and Dietetics.

CQI Programs

A continuous quality improvement program (CQI) program is very important and offers many benefits. The first and probably most important benefit is improved patient outcomes. This can occur by identifying patients who are having trouble as well as identifying programs or protocols that are not effective. A CQI program also offers the benefit of patient safety because protocols provide standardized care that has been proven through research. It helps to prevent errors from occurring as well. All practitioners follow the same guidelines, which is extremely helpful when people are busy. It also lessens the chance for variability in treatments and should eliminate judgment calls. CQI programs should also help increase patient satisfaction because care is optimized, and the benefits to the patient would include increased quality of life and decreased rate of hospitalization. CQI programs should also help to control costs and reduce the amount of waste. The program also helps with documentation, which should enable enhanced reimbursement from the Centers for Medicare and Medicaid Services (CMS).

CQI for Anemia Management

First, the committee in charge of developing the CQI program should review trends of the patients in that facility such as ferritin or hemoglobin levels or those not responsive to erythropoietin (EPO) therapy because of iron deficiency. The literature should be reviewed. It is helpful to review any published standards of care such as the NKF K/DOQI guidelines. The next step may be to review the IV iron therapy that is currently used and to decide if changing to a different product might be a way to address low response to EPO therapy. Following a review of current practice in that facility, the results should be compared to K/DOQI recommendations especially for target laboratory values such as ferritin, serum transferrin saturation (TSAT), or hemoglobin. Next, education should be completed with all staff involved in this process to make sure they understand how to manage anemia, how to provide IV iron, and how to assess for infection or inflammation. After all this is accomplished, implementation can occur.

Evaluating CQI for Anemia Management

The final outcome of the CQI program should be improving patient outcomes and reaching target levels for hemoglobin, serum transferrin saturation (TSAT), and/or ferritin. Standardizing the provision of erythropoietin (EPO) and iron including dosages and product selection is also a possible outcome. This should also help to reduce common errors in anemia management. Patient trends should also be noted and any variation in the trend examined. For example, perhaps a positive trend in ferritin or hemoglobin level was noticed after the type of iron preparation was changed. This would be a positive outcome for the CQI program. After trends of all patients are examined, then individual patients not meeting goals can be addressed further. Additionally, the various parts of the program are evaluated, and all practitioners involved, such as the dietitian, nurse, and physician, are responsible for reporting on their individual area of expertise.

Adult Patients with Bone Disease and CKD

There are many potential outcome indicators that can be used for a CQI program for monitoring bone disease in adult patients with CKD. These may include:

- The percent of patients with parathyroid hormone with a target range of 35-70 pg/mL for Stage 3, 70-110 pg/mL for Stage 4, and 150- 300 pg/mL for Stage 5 CKD
- The percent of patients with serum phosphorus between 2.7- 4.6 mg/dL for patients with Stage 3 or 4 CKD
- The percent of patients with serum phosphorus between 3.5-5.5 mg/dL for patients with Stage 5 CKD.
- The percent of patients who have received dietary instruction on low phosphorus diet from a registered dietitian
- The percent of patients who are prescribed phosphate binders after implementation of a dietary phosphorus restriction with a parathyroid hormone level that remains outside the designated target range
- The percent of patients with hypercalcemia (serum calcium greater than 10.2 mg/dL)
- For patients receiving phosphate binders and who are hypercalcemic, the percent of patients who are receiving a non-calcium–based phosphate binder

Patients with Diabetes and CKD

There are many potential outcome indicators that can be used for a CQI program for patients with diabetes and CKD. These may include:

- The percent of patients with a **HbA_{1c}** (glycosylated hemoglobin) that is within the target of less than 7%
- The percent of patients with a blood pressure reading meeting the target range of less than 130/80 mm Hg
- The percentage of patients with diabetes and hypertension with Stage 1-4 CKD whoa re treated with an ACE inhibitor
- The percentage of patients who have received medical nutrition therapy to address diabetes and CKD
- The percentage of patients who have self-management skills documented in the medical record
- The percentage of patients with an LDL level less than 100 mg/dL
- For those patients with LDL greater than 100 mg/dL, the percentage that have had a statin prescribed to treat

Patients with Dyslipidemia and CKD

There are many potential outcome indicators that can be used for a CQI program for managing dyslipidemia and CKD. These may include:

- The percentage of adults and adolescents who have been screened for dyslipidemia including a fasting lipid profile, HDL, LDL, and triglyceride levels
- The percentage of these patients who were fasting the night before the lipid profile was drawn
- The percentage of adult patients who had a triglyceride level greater than 500 mg/dL who had a triglyceride-lowering agent prescribed using a fibrate or nicotinic acid medication
- The percentage of patients who have had dietary instruction with a registered dietitian for instituting the Therapeutic Lifestyle Changes (TLC) diet
- The percentage of patients receiving cyclosporine with an elevated LDL level who have been prescribed a statin medication

Laboratory Data for Assessing Nutrition and CKD

There are many potential outcome indicators using laboratory data for a CQI program for assessing nutrition and CKD. These may include:

- The percentage of hemodialysis patients who have had a predialysis serum albumin level drawn monthly
- The percentage of patients with a serum albumin level greater than 4 g/dL
- The percentage of patients with a predialysis serum creatinine less than 10 mg/dL who have received nutrition assessment for protein energy malnutrition
- The percentage of patients who have a predialysis serum cholesterol level less than 180 mg/dL who have received documented nutrition assessment by a registered dietitian
- The percentage of patients who have had the protein catabolic rate calculated and documented monthly

Nonlaboratory Data for CKD

There are many potential outcome indicators using nonlaboratory measures that can be used for a CQI program for assessing nutrition and CKD. These may include:

- The percentage of patients who have received a monthly measure of current body weight compared to usual postdialysis weight
- The percentage of patients who have received documentation of subjective global assessment (SGA) at least every 6 months
- The percentage of patients who have received a detailed dietary recall or interview or evaluation of food records at least every 6 months

- The percentage of patients who have had their edema-free body weight readjusted based on postdialysis weight. Those with an edema-free body weight between 95%-115% of the NHANES II median standard will have their actual weight used for calculations. For those above 115% or below 95%, an adjusted edema-free body weight will be used for calculations

Serum Phosphorus, Calcium, and PTH

Possible outcome indicators for children with various stages of CKD using serum calcium, phosphorus, and parathyroid hormone (PTH) level are as follows:

- The percentage of children with Stage 2 CKD who have their serum calcium, phosphorus, and PTH level checked at least yearly
- The percentage of children with Stage 3 CKD who have these levels checked at least every 6 months
- The percentage of children with Stage 4 CKD who have these levels checked at least every 3 months
- The percentage of children with stage 5 CKD who have serum calcium and phosphorus checked monthly and PTH level checked at least every 3 months
- The percentage of children with a target level for PTH for stage 2 and 3 CKD is 35-70 pg/mL, for stage 4 is 70-110 pg/mL, and for stage 5 is 200-300 pg/mL

Assessing Bone Status for Children with CKD

Possible outcome indicators are as follows:

- The percentage of children with stage 5 CKD who receive a bone biopsy for suspected bone fracture
- The percentage of children with stage 5 CKD who are suspected of having aluminum toxicity or who have a history of aluminum exposure who receive a bone biopsy
- The percentage of children with stage 5 CKD who have a chronically elevated serum calcium level greater than 400 pg/mL who receive a bone biopsy
- The percentage of children with CKD who receive a bone biopsy when rickets or symptomatic proximal slipped epiphyses are suspected or to evaluate the maturation of the skeleton

Target Phosphorus Levels

Possible outcome indicators for children with CKD using target phosphorus levels are as follows:

- The percentage of children with stage 1-4 CKD who have a serum phosphorus in the target range of 4.5-6.5 mg/dL for ages 1-5 years, 3.6-5.8 mg/dL for ages 6-12, and 2.3-4.5 mg/dL for ages 13-20
- The percentage of children whose serum phosphorus is above the target range and who have a dietary phosphorus restriction implemented at the level of the Dietary Reference Intake (DRI) for the following age ranges:

- less than 6 months = 100 mg per day
- 6 months to 1 year = 275 mg
- 3 years = 460 mg
- 4-8 years = 500 mg
- 9-18 years = 1250 mg
- The percentage of children with serum phosphorus levels above the target range and who are following a phosphorus restricted diet who start phosphate binder therapy
- The percentage of children who are starting phosphate binders who receive a calcium-based phosphate binder as initial therapy

Vitamin D Levels

Possible outcome indicators are as follows:

- The percentage of children with CKD and a parathyroid hormone (PTH) level above the target range who have a serum 25-hydroxy vitamin D level checked
- The percentage of children with a serum 25-hydroxy vitamin D level less than 30 ng/mL who begin supplementation with ergocalciferol (vitamin D2)
- The percentage of children receiving ergocalciferol who have a serum calcium and phosphorus level drawn after 1 month then at least every 3 months
- The percentage of children receiving ergocalciferol who have this withheld if serum calcium levels are greater than 10.2 mg/dL
- The percentage of children with stage 5 CKD who begin calcitriol therapy for PTH level greater than 300 pg/mL
- The percentage of children receiving calcitriol therapy who have their doses adjusted by 50% if the serum PTH level is not reduced by 30% after 3 months of therapy, if the serum calcium and phosphorus are within target ranges

Development and Assessment of Nutrition Prescription

Nutrition Screening

Nutrition screening is a process utilized to identify individuals who are malnourished or who have risk factors for developing malnutrition. These individuals would then be identified as requiring a full nutrition assessment. The overall goal is to improve patient care and overall medical outcomes. For hospitalized patients, the Joint Commission on Hospital Accreditation requires that nutrition screening be completed within 24 hours of admission to the hospital. There are many factors that can be used in the screening process. These include changes in usual weight, weight status, type of diagnosis, past medical history that may impact nutritional status, requirement of a specialized diet, use of enteral or parenteral nutrition, and certain laboratory data such as albumin. Other types of information that may be obtained include diet history, functional status, social issues, gastrointestinal function, ability to chew and swallow adequately, and medication use.

Nutrition Assessment and MNT

Nutrition assessment is the process utilized by a registered dietitian (RD) that uses information pertaining to diet, weight status and history, medical history, physical exam, social history, medication use, and laboratory data to provide an estimation of the individual's nutritional status. Information obtained from the nutrition screen is also utilized. Medical nutrition therapy (MNT) involves nutrition screening and nutrition assessment as well as the treatment component that may involve specialized diet therapy, nutrition support, or nutrition and diet education. The Academy of Nutrition and Dietetics describes MNT as "an essential component of comprehensive health services." MNT is part of the Medicare Reform Act involving preventative care and managing certain chronic diseases.

Comprehensive Information

The information derived from obtaining an individual's diet history should be comprehensive. This information is generally a synopsis of the individual's usual diet and meal patterns. Basic financial information should be obtained to evaluate whether there are any financial obstacles to obtaining food. Information about family and household should be obtained, such as who shops and prepares the meals, and the presence of adequate food storage and preparation equipment. Information on appetite, food allergies or intolerances, or religious factors affecting food choices should be obtained. Determining oral or dental factors that may impact nutritional status is required, as well as any gastrointestinal issues such as nausea, vomiting, or changes in bowel habits. Information about the impact of any chronic diseases on food intake or diet should be noted along with medication use and vitamin, mineral, or herbal supplements. Any other pertinent information should also be obtained, such as the presence of certain attitudes, beliefs, or misinformation about diet or food that may impact nutritional status.

Diet History and Disadvantages

Nutrient intake analysis is a tool used to calculate actual intake of food either through direct observation or by calculating what is left on a tray to determine what was actually consumed. This is also known as a calorie count. The data for this type of analysis should be gathered for at least 72 hours. The desired nutrient analysis is then calculated and documented appropriately. A food record (also called a food diary) is a similar tool but is typically used in an outpatient setting. Data is collected over a period of time, typically 3-7 days and the food consumed is recorded as it is eaten. Once the food record is completed, the desired nutrient analysis is calculated. The nutrient analysis results obtained from either tool is typically compared to the dietary reference intakes (DRIs) or to the USDA's MyPlate. The disadvantages include the following: possible inaccuracies in recording or estimating portion sizes, the need for the individual to be literate, and the possibility that the information may be subjective.

Food Frequency and 24-Hour Recall

The food frequency is a questionnaire used to obtain information from an individual regarding how often certain foods are consumed on a daily, weekly, or monthly basis. It is a method that utilizes retrospective information, thus relies on memory. This method does not identify specific nutrient deficiencies but instead identifies general food groups that may be missing from an individual's diet. A food frequency is often more useful when used in conjunction with the individual's usual intake. A 24-hour recall is another method to collect information on an individual's diet that utilizes memory of what was consumed in the previous 24 hours. Once the information is collected, the desired nutrient analysis is calculated. Disadvantages to this method are inaccuracy of memory and inability to estimate portion sizes. Another disadvantage is overestimating or underestimating the amount of food actually consumed. A combination of the various methods is often employed as a way to get a better idea of an individual's typical diet.

ARF Patients

Metabolic Alterations

There are many metabolic alterations that are possible in a patient with acute renal failure (ARF). These changes can be further compounded by a catabolic state associated with critical illness, type of treatment, and other underlying medical issues. Hyperglycemia is one such alteration that may occur. This can be due to changes in peripheral insulin resistance and a reduction of glucose uptake by skeletal muscles. The presence of diabetes or the use of corticosteroid medications will further compound this issue. The potential implications of elevated blood glucose levels are multifactorial. They can affect a patient's ability to wean from mechanical ventilation. Hyperglycemia also increases the risk for infection and for poor wound healing. Hyperglycemia can also lead to issues with fluid balance as dehydration, hypernatremia, or hyperosmolar coma.

Protein and Lipid Metabolism

The rate of protein metabolism is markedly increased in patients with ARF. This is due in part to ARF and can be exacerbated by starvation. Insulin resistance is responsible for the increased rate of muscle metabolism. Increases in parathyroid hormone can also increase protein metabolism. This accelerated rate of protein metabolism, known as catabolism, will not be affected by providing increased nutrient intake. The implications of protein catabolism include alterations in immune function and delayed wound healing. Alterations in lipid metabolism can also occur due to changes in lipolysis. There is a reduction in the activity of lipoprotein lipase and hepatic triglyceride lipase. Insulin resistance also plays a role. Levels of total cholesterol and HDL cholesterol will be decreased. Triglyceride and LDL cholesterol levels may be increased.

Medical Nutrition Therapy

Medical nutrition therapy for the adult patient with ARF should be based on an individual's clinical status, laboratory data, fluid balance, and type of dialysis being provided. Continued reassessment is crucial as clinical status can change quickly. The amount of protein required during ARF is still under debate; however, a protein intake less than 0.8 g/kg (the RDA) is not recommended. Those patients receiving renal replacement therapy should receive between 1.2-1.5 g of protein/kg to account for losses. Fluid requirements are generally assessed by determining 24-hour urine output then adding an additional 500 mL per day. Additional increases may be necessary during diuresis, fever, or sepsis, or if the patient is receiving continuous renal replacement therapy (CRRT). Sodium is usually restricted to 2-3 g per day. Potassium is typically restricted to 2-3 g per day and is dependent on serum potassium level and dialysis. Phosphorus is typically restricted to approximately 8-15 mg/kg. This is affected by the use of phosphorus binders, changes in renal function, and dialysis schedule.

Energy Requirements

Calorie requirements are estimated to be 25-35 kcal/kg or 20%-30% above basal energy expenditure (BEE). ARF does not directly increase energy requirements; however, the presence of sepsis or multiorgan failure can increase requirements. Current recommendations call for the use of ideal body weight in the calculation of energy requirements, but the efficacy of this practice remains under debate. The use of actual weight or usual weight may be a better practice to prevent over- or under-feeding for those who are morbidly obese, significantly underweight, or who have amputations. Overfeeding is dangerous because it can cause fatty liver, increased body temperature, and carbon dioxide retention that can adversely affect a patient's ability to wean from the ventilator. Underfeeding is not recommended as it may increase protein catabolism or worsen nitrogen balance; however, the effects of underfeeding are less of a risk than overfeeding.

Oral Diet and Tube Feedings

An oral diet is always preferred over tube feeding or parenteral nutrition. Sometimes, conditions may not allow an oral diet to be implemented. Patients who are critically ill and in the intensive care unit are often unable to take an oral diet. This is further compounded by the presence of a mechanical ventilator or intensive treatments that would interfere with meals. Oftentimes, the patient is physically unable to eat or needs significant assistance. For those patients who are able to eat an oral diet, nutrition supplements are often offered to help improve intake. Tube feedings can also be used either alone or in combination with an oral diet. Products are available that contain essential amino acids or are designed for hemodialysis patients. Whatever product is selected should be carefully evaluated to meet the patient's nutrient and fluid requirements. Consideration must be given to the tube-feeding rate based on the other treatments that are involved, or the tube feeding may be excessively held and not provide adequate nutrition.

TPN

The main consideration for initiating total parenteral nutrition (TPN) is the type of renal replacement therapy the patient is receiving. The goal of TPN is to reduce protein catabolism and to try to minimize urea production without increasing the dialysis requirement. Although solutions containing only essential amino acids are available, a mix of essential and nonessential amino acids is recommended. Lipids should be provided as a substrate in part to help reduce the respiratory quotient and to reduce excessive amounts of calories from dextrose. A lower glucose load may be indicated if the patient begins to experience hyperglycemia. Additionally, some dextrose may be absorbed from certain types of continuous renal replacement therapy (CRRT). Electrolytes should be adjusted based on laboratory data. The use of TPN to control electrolyte abnormalities is not recommended. Fluid allowance is based on urine output, fluid balance, clinical condition, and type of renal replacement therapy. Concentrated forms of substrates may be used instead, such as 70% dextrose concentration.

Medical Nutrition Therapy

Monitoring a patient with ARF is consistent with monitoring patients with other types of disease states. Initial monitoring of glucose, phosphorus, and potassium is important due to the potential for shifts related to refeeding syndrome. BUN level should be monitored as a way to gauge protein intake. Electrolytes should be checked twice per day in patients who are somewhat stable, more often for those who are unstable. Patients who are unstable may require serum glucose and potassium levels to be drawn every 2- 4 hours. Bilirubin, ammonia, and liver function tests should be monitored twice per week until the patient is stable, and then should be monitored weekly. Accurate intake and output records should be kept, and caloric intake should be calculated daily. The overall nutrition plan will need constant readjustment to respond to changes in clinical status. This is best accomplished by a registered dietitian.

ESRD Patient

Goals for Medical Nutrition Therapy

The main goal of medical nutrition therapy for the end stage renal disease (ESRD) patient is to prevent malnutrition. For both adults and children, this means maintaining a good nutritional status, and for children, maintaining normal growth and development. This encompasses the adequate provision of nutrients such as protein, calories, vitamins, and minerals. Other goals include regulating fluid and electrolyte imbalance. Preventing the development of bone issues such as renal osteodystrophy is another goal. This involves appropriate intake of calcium, phosphorus, and vitamin D. It is important to allow the individual to consume a diet that is nutritionally sound and appropriate for the disease state while being attractive and pleasing. This diet should also be able to be incorporated into the individual's lifestyle without too much fuss or trouble. Because long-term patients will be in control of their diet and treatment, education early on is essential.

Dialysis Patients

Protein Requirements for Infants and Children (Predialysis Stage)

The estimated protein requirements in infants, children, and adolescents are as follows:

Age 0 – 6 months = 2.2 g/kg body weight
Age 6 – 12 months = 2 g/ kg body weight
Age 1 – 3 years = 0.18 g/cm height
Age 4 – 6 years = 0.21 g/cm height
Age 7 – 10 years = 0.21 g/cm height
Age 11 – 14 years = 0.29 g/cm height
Age 15 – 18 years = 0.34 g/cm height

Protein Requirements for Infants and Children

Infants birth to 6 months receiving hemodialysis, protein intake is estimated at 2.6 g/kg and for 7 months to 1 year, 2.0 g/kg. For children receiving hemodialysis, protein intake should be in the range of 1.6 g/kg for ages 4-6 and 1.4 g/kg for ages up to age 14. For ages 15-18 years, protein recommendations are 1.2-1.3 g/ kg. Protein requirements for children on continuous ambulatory peritoneal dialysis (CAPD) are based on the recommended dietary allowance (RDA) plus an additional factor to cover losses. For infants up to 6 months receiving CAPD, protein recommendations are 2.9-3.0 g/kg, and for 7 months to 1 year, 2.3-2.4 g/kg. Children receiving CAPD up to the age of 6 years may require 1.9-2.0 g/kg. Children 7-10 years receiving CAPD may require 1.7-1.8 g/kg, age 11-14 years may require 1.2-1.3 g/ kg, and for those children over the age of 14, 1.4-1.5 g/ kg. Urea kinetic modeling can be done for children in positive nitrogen balance to get a more accurate estimation of protein requirements.

Patient Guidelines

K/DOQI guidelines have been established for adult hemodialysis patients. Calorie requirements are estimated to be approximately 35 kcal/kg. For adults who are older than 60 or who are obese, calorie requirements may be slightly lower at 30 kcal/kg. This lower level takes into account a less active lifestyle and a lower amount of lean body mass. Calorie requirements may also be higher for underweight individuals or for those who have a very active lifestyle. Potassium allowance is based on the amount of urine output. Approximately 2-2.5 g/day is generally a reasonable level unless the patient is anuric. Sodium and fluid allowances are interrelated and based on fluid balance, blood pressure, and remaining residual kidney function. If the patient's fluid output is more than 1 liter per day, an allowance of 2-4 g/day of sodium with 2 liters of fluid is appropriate. If output is less than 1 liter per day, a restriction of 2 g of sodium and 1-1.5 liters of fluid per day may be warranted.

Patient Protein Intake

The K/DOQI guidelines suggest that adult hemodialysis patients should consume 1.2 g per kg of protein per day. Adult patients receiving peritoneal dialysis should consume 1.2-1.3 g per kg. The protein should consist of at least 50% high biological value, such as meat, chicken, fish, eggs, soy protein, and dairy. The protein allowance is at this level because of the amount of protein that can be lost in the dialysate during each treatment. Implications of protein deficiency include poor wound healing, fluid imbalance, and impaired immune function. Consuming adequate protein will also help to maintain normal serum albumin levels. Low serum albumin has been associated with inflammation and in turn can increase the morbidity and mortality risk.

Calcium, Phosphorus, and Vitamin D for Adult Patients

Calcium requirements for the adult hemodialysis patient are individualized and largely based on intake through the diet, use of calcium supplements and phosphate binders, and level of vitamin D intake. It is also based on laboratory data and the amount of calcium used in the dialysate. Dietary calcium intake is typically restricted because phosphorus is restricted in the diet, which concurrently limits calcium intake. For patients with hypocalcemia, calcium supplements are generally implemented and the amount of calcium in the dialysate is adjusted. According to the NKF K/DOQI guidelines, phosphorus intake is usually restricted if the glomerular filtration rate (GFR) is less than 60 mL/min/1.73 m2. A typical restriction is 800-1000 mg per day. The use of phosphate binders may also be warranted. Vitamin D is required in the biologically active form at a level of 5-15 μg/day taken under the supervision of a physician specializing in nephrology.

Energy Requirements for Adolescents

Energy requirements for an adolescent receiving hemodialysis are based on age and gender. Boys 11-14 years will require approximately 55 kcal/kg and those 15-18 years will require 45 kcal/kg. Girls 11-14 years will require 47 kcal/kg and those 15-18 years will require 40 kcal/kg. Sodium is generally restricted to 2-4 g/day if the child is anuric, has elevated blood pressure, or has significant fluid retention. Fluid is calculated by considering insensible losses, amount of urine output, and other losses along with the ultrafiltration capacity. Acceptable intradialytic weight gain for an adolescent is approximately 1.5-2 kg for 3-day intervals. Potassium is restricted for adolescents with elevated serum potassium levels, and the typical restriction is 2-4 g/day. Calcium should be provided at 100% of the dietary reference intake. Phosphorus is typically restricted to less than 800 mg/day. Vitamin D is prescribed based on parathyroid hormone, calcium, and phosphorus levels.

Calorie Requirements for the Adult Patient

For patients younger than age 60, 35 kcal/kg is recommended. This level is sufficient to maintain positive nitrogen balance and maintain weight. For patients over the age of 60, 30 kcal/kg is recommended. For PD patients with a lower activity level or lower amounts of lean body mass, 30 kcal/kg is the goal. One consideration to take into account when determining caloric intake is the amount of glucose that is absorbed from the dialysate. Patients on PD can absorb as much as 33% of their calorie requirements from the dialysate itself. There are many formulas that can be used to estimate the amount of glucose that is absorbed. One formula is to assume that 60% of the glucose is absorbed. For a 1-liter bag of 2.5% dextrose, 85 kcals of dextrose are available. 60% of this number is 51 kcals, the amount absorbed.

General Nutrient Guidelines

The general guidelines for nutrient intake for the adult PD patient are typically liberal due to the nature of PD. The protein allowance is estimated at 1.2-1.3 g/kg, although more may be indicated if the patient has peritonitis or is malnourished. Sodium is not typically restricted as sodium is easily removed by PD. Potassium is also easily removed by PD, and most patients will not require a potassium restriction. In certain cases, some patients may actually require potassium supplementation for low serum levels. Calcium is generally limited to less than 2000 mg/day and the majority of this is from calcium-based phosphate binders. A restriction of 800-1000 mg of phosphorus is usually required; however, this is difficult to maintain because of the higher protein requirements. Phosphate binders are often used to help control phosphorus levels. Fluids are not typically restricted because fluid balance is titrated using differing dextrose concentrations of the dialysate.

Oral Supplements

There are many supplements available for use in patients who are not eating properly and require caloric and other nutrient supplementation. Some are designed specifically for patients with renal disease and others are not. Products such as Suplena, Nepro, Magnacal Renal, Nutra-Renal, or Renalcal are designed for patients with impaired kidney function. These products are calorically dense at 2 kcal/mL, and have low to moderate amounts of protein depending upon the product and its designated use. Sodium and potassium content are reduced to help with electrolyte control. Phosphorus content is also limited. Other products such as milkshakes, Instant Breakfast drinks, or standard enteral formulas are not designed for individuals with kidney disease. The protein, electrolyte, and fluid content may not be appropriate for all patients. Other products that are fluid restricted, such as Nutren 2.0 or Boost Plus, may be useful in some patients but are not low in electrolytes, which may cause an issue for those with unstable electrolytes.

CKD

Enteral Feedings

One of the main considerations for initiating enteral feedings in a patient with CKD is malnutrition, which is commonly seen in patients with CKD and can increase the risk for death or other complications. Tube feedings are a safe way to deliver additional nutrition. The issues that need to be considered are energy and protein requirements, fluid balance, and laboratory data. The condition of the GI tract is also important. A formula should be selected that most closely meets the needs of the patient. The type of formula selected may include renal, standard, fluid-restricted, elemental- or peptide-based, or fiber-containing formulations. Sometimes a modular product such as protein powder will need to be added to more closely meet a patient's nutrient requirements. Cost may be an issue as the more specialized a formulation is, the more expensive it will be. Additionally, renal formulations generally have a higher osmolarity than standard formulations.

Options for the Administration of Enteral Feedings

There are a few options for managing the enteral feeding administration in a patient with CKD. The decision should be based on the individual patient's needs such as clinical status or the need for time away from the enteral feeding pump. Continuous feedings are often used for the initial tube feeding. Often times the patient is ill and hospitalized and this type of schedule is useful in this scenario. Cyclic feedings are often used as a way to transition from tube feedings to an oral diet. The feedings can be provided at night then stopped a few hours prior to breakfast. Intermittent feedings are another type of schedule that can be used to allow a patient a break from the pump during certain times of the day. The feedings can be scheduled around mealtime to be more physiologic in nature. The actual schedule will depend upon the patient's tolerance of the bolus type feedings and nutrient requirements.

Hyperglycemia in Tube-Fed Patients

At least 66% of patients with CKD have either Type 1 or Type 2 diabetes. This factor alone can contribute to hyperglycemia being a fairly common complication of tube feedings. Patients with CKD have issues with peripheral insulin resistance and reduced clearance of insulin, which can cause hyperglycemia. These factors can be further exacerbated by acute illness. Critically ill patients also experience an increase in gluconeogenesis, which can worsen hyperglycemia. Absorption of the dextrose concentration in the dialysate is another factor that contributes to hyperglycemia. Certain types of medications such as corticosteroids can contribute to hyperglycemia. The short- term consequences of hyperglycemia in an acutely ill patient with CKD are delayed wound healing, increased chance of infection, and the development of diabetic ketoacidosis. Treating hyperglycemia involves providing subcutaneous insulin at a reduced level of usual requirements supplemented with a sliding scale schedule. Alternatively, an insulin drip can be utilized. Oral hypoglycemic agents can also be used for those patients who are not critically or acutely ill.

Diarrhea in Tube-Fed Patients

Diarrhea is a very common complication of tube feedings especially in acutely ill patients. There are many potential reasons for diarrhea including medications with high osmolarity or as an elixir containing sorbitol, which can cause an osmotic-type diarrhea. Antibiotics can also cause diarrhea because they affect normal gut flora that can lead to diarrhea. Other potential causes include hyperosmolar formulas that are commonly seen in formulations designed for renal dysfunction, administration of cold formula, or too rapid an administration of a formula. Gastrointestinal dysmotility can also be a cause as well as hypoalbuminemia, which are common in patients with chronic kidney disease (CKD). A review of medications, the use of soluble fiber, and a careful review of the tube-feeding plan should all be considered as part of the treatment plan. Certain types of antidiarrheal agents can be used such as Lomotil or Kaopectate. The use of any other type of medication needs to be carefully considered in relation to CKD.

Clogged Feeding Tubes

The most common cause of clogged feeding tubes in any patient is improper administration of medications through the feeding tube. Because of this, the liquid form of medication should be considered if possible, to help prevent clogging. Acidic type medications need to be diluted before being given to the patient as these may cause the formula to curdle in the stomach causing the tube to clog. A pharmacist should be available for consult to make sure the medications are being given appropriately, at the correct dose for the patient, and in the correct form. Warm water flushes are typically the best method for maintaining the patency of the feeding tube. Cranberry juice and cola have been used, but there is no evidence that these types of fluids work any better. The main concern for flushing a tube is the amount of fluid the patient can tolerate, as many patients with CKD require fluid restriction. Frequent flushes add volume; therefore, the medication schedule should be closely reviewed to achieve the most efficient schedule possible for the patient.

TPN

As part of the nutrition assessment of a patient with CKD being considered for nutrition support, the indications and contraindications for total parenteral nutrition (TPN) should be considered. An indication for TPN would be a nonfunctioning GI tract. The route of administration (central versus peripheral) needs to be considered as the patient may not be a good candidate for central line placement and may not be able to handle the large volumes often required with the peripheral route. Fluid requirement is important, as many patients with CKD require volume restriction. Electrolyte management is also important as patients with CKD often have metabolic abnormalities that may worsen with TPN. The overall goal of nutrition support is also important and should be determined in conjunction with the patient's prognosis.

TPN Initiation and Discontinuation

Generally, TPN can be initiated with full amino acid allotment but with a reduced calorie intake of approximately 1000 kcals. This is to help reduce the risk of refeeding. It also lets the nutrition support practitioner monitor for adverse effects of any of the TPN components. Often, volume is initially restricted to 1000 mL per day. If tolerated, the TPN volume can be advanced along with calories and electrolytes. If there are any signs of laboratory abnormalities such as hyperglycemia, these should be addressed before the TPN is advanced. TPN can begin to be weaned when the patient is able to meet approximately 60% of calorie requirements through either tube feedings or an oral diet. TPN should not be abruptly stopped to prevent rebound hypoglycemia. The rate should be reduced by 50% 1-2 hours prior to stopping the TPN. If the TPN needs to be stopped quickly because the line has been lost or some other reason, providing 10% dextrose via IV at half the TPN rate is an option to help with blood glucose control.

TPN Monitoring

Guidelines for monitoring TPN are dependent upon the clinical status of the patient. Sicker, more unstable patients require more frequent monitoring. Daily monitoring of weight, intake and output, subjective global assessment, and appetite if the patient is eating is required. Blood urea nitrogen (BUN), electrolytes, calcium, phosphorus, and magnesium should be monitored daily until stable, and then can be monitored 2-3 times per week. Serum glucose often requires monitoring as many as 4-6 times per day until stable. More frequent checks may be required for those in the intensive care unit (ICU) receiving continuous insulin infusion. Triglycerides should be checked on initiation of TPN, then every week. Liver function tests and serum bilirubin should also be checked on initiation, then monitored weekly. Complete blood count (CBC) should be monitored every day until stable, then can be monitored 2-3 times per week. Serum albumin, prealbumin, or other hepatic proteins should be monitored weekly.

Dextrose

The main calorie source for TPN is dextrose monohydrate. This provides 3.4 kcal/gram. It is available in 50% and 70% solutions for use in TPN. All sources of dextrose need to be taken into account including intravenous fluids, medications, and dialysate when determining the dextrose prescription for TPN. Total glucose intake should be limited to 3-5 mg/kg/minute for optimal glucose control. Adverse effects of excessive glucose administration include elevated blood glucose, increased carbon dioxide production and subsequent difficulty weaning from the ventilator, lipogenesis, and liver complications such as steatosis or cholestasis. Too much carbohydrate can also affect immune function. Insulin is usually required to help control blood glucose levels in patients with chronic kidney disease (CKD) receiving

TPN, especially if the patient has preexisting diabetes. A goal of 100-150 mg/dL is reasonable.

Lipids

Lipids are used as an energy source in TPN. They typically provide 20%-30% of total calories. For peripheral solutions, up to 60% of total calories can be provided. Lipids are low in osmolarity. Lipids also provide a source of essential fatty acids with 2%-4% of total calories required to prevent essential fatty acid deficiency. Lipids are a component of propofol and need to be accounted for in patients receiving both TPN and propofol. Adverse effects of lipids include hyperlipidemia and immune system suppression. Triglyceride levels should be monitored and lipids held if the level is greater than 400 mg/dL. Additionally, patients with egg allergy should not receive lipids because they contain egg phospholipid.

Amino Acids

Amino acids should be provided as a mixture of both essential and nonessential amino acids. In the past, just essential amino acids were provided; however, there is no data to support this practice. The amount of amino acids required is dependent upon the stage of kidney disease and the mode of dialysis. For pre-dialysis patients, amino acids should be limited to 0.6-1.0 g/kg/day. For those receiving chronic dialysis (peritoneal or hemodialysis), 1.2-1.3 g/kg should be provided. Patients receiving continuous renal replacement therapy require a minimum of 1.0 g/kg and may require as much as 2.5 g/kg depending upon losses and overall clinical condition. Provision of too much amino acid in the TPN solution can affect renal function and dialysis requirements.

Acid-Base Balance

Acid-base balance can be difficult to manage in patients with CKD but can be addressed somewhat with the use of TPN. Sodium bicarbonate can be given through an intravenous line. Bicarbonate is not used in TPN solutions because it can bind with calcium and magnesium to form an insoluble salt. Instead, acetate is used. Acetate is metabolized by the liver into bicarbonate. Metabolic acidosis can occur when the glomerular filtration rate falls below 25%. If the patient is experiencing metabolic acidosis, more acetate than chloride is provided. If the patient is experiencing metabolic alkalosis, then more chloride is provided. The amounts of either should be adjusted daily until the appropriate acid-base balance is achieved. This is determined by the serum bicarbonate and chloride levels.

Electrolytes

Serum magnesium, phosphorus, and potassium levels may be difficult to control with TPN. These levels tend to rise as kidney function worsens. Serum potassium, phosphorus, and magnesium may be adversely affected by refeeding if the patient was malnourished or without nutrition for a significant length of time before starting TPN. The nutritional status of the patient needs to be taken into account when ordering the electrolyte prescription. Phosphorus is not efficiently dialyzed; therefore, a reduced level of phosphate in the TPN solution is usually required but possibly not initially. Serum sodium is sometimes difficult to control as well. Serum sodium measures hydration. Fluid losses as well as sodium losses will affect serum levels. Sodium requirements may range from 40-60 mEq/L of solution. Potassium requirements may be 10-40 mEq/L of solution. Phosphorus requirements may be 5-10 mmol/L and magnesium requirements may be 5-10 mEq/L.

PPN

Peripheral parenteral nutrition (PPN) has many limitations. The use of PPN is limited to 2 weeks or less. Because it is infused in a smaller peripheral vein rather than a large central vein, access is often difficult to obtain. For this same reason, the osmolarity of the solution must be less than 900 mOsm/L to help protect the vein. This limit on the osmolarity also limits the amount of dextrose and amino acids that can be provided, as these two components significantly contribute to osmolarity. Lipids can be given at 50%-60% of total calories, but many patients on dialysis have an inflammatory process occurring and require lipids to be restricted to less than 30% of total calories. Additionally, up to 3 liters of PPN per day are often required to attain the appropriate osmolarity, and patients with CKD cannot handle this volume, making it difficult to meet full nutrient requirements. Because the disadvantages of PPN outweigh advantages, its use is not usually recommended for patients with CKD.

Children with CKD

Nutrition Care Plan for a Child with CKD

There are several components that need to be evaluated in order to develop a thorough nutrition care plan. The first is assessment of growth using standardized procedures such as recumbent length, weight, head circumference, and triceps skinfold measurements, comparing these measurements to reference data. A dietary interview is necessary that captures such information as regular intake, and changes in appetite, intake, or social situation. Actual intake is assessed compared to estimated requirements. A complete medical history is required, including medication use, laboratory data, blood pressure, and information on bowel habits. Additionally, information regarding the consumption of non-food items such as paper is also important. Information regarding fluid balance, ability to feed self, as well as the overall appearance of the child should be obtained. This would include the appearance of the hair, skin, mouth, and other parts of the body. Finally, information regarding the child's psychosocial history is also important.

Energy Requirements for Children Receiving Maintenance Dialysis

The starting point for calculating energy requirements for children should be the Recommended Dietary Allowance (RDA) for chronological age. The RDAs for children are as follows:

- Birth to 6 months= 108 kcal/kg
- 6 months to 1 year= 98 kcal/kg
- 1-3 years= 102 kcal/kg

- 4-6 years= 90 kcal/kg
- 7-10 years= 70 kcal/kg
- for males 11-14 years= 55 kcal/kg; 15-18 years= 45 kcal/kg; 18-21 years= 40 kcal/kg
- for females 11-14 years= 47 kcal/kg; 15-18 years= 40 kcal/kg; 18-21 years= 38 kcal/kg

The adequacy of caloric intake must be reassessed and adjusted accordingly. Children who are malnourished and underweight may require additional calories for catch-up growth to occur. Additionally, indirect calorimetry can be done to calculate resting energy expenditure to compare to the RDA.

How to Overcome Test Anxiety

Just the thought of taking a test is enough to make most people a little nervous. A test is an important event that can have a long-term impact on your future, so it's important to take it seriously and it's natural to feel anxious about performing well. But just because anxiety is normal, that doesn't mean that it's helpful in test taking, or that you should simply accept it as part of your life. Anxiety can have a variety of effects. These effects can be mild, like making you feel slightly nervous, or severe, like blocking your ability to focus or remember even a simple detail.

If you experience test anxiety—whether severe or mild—it's important to know how to beat it. To discover this, first you need to understand what causes test anxiety.

Causes of Test Anxiety

While we often think of anxiety as an uncontrollable emotional state, it can actually be caused by simple, practical things. One of the most common causes of test anxiety is that a person does not feel adequately prepared for their test. This feeling can be the result of many different issues such as poor study habits or lack of organization, but the most common culprit is time management. Starting to study too late, failing to organize your study time to cover all of the material, or being distracted while you study will mean that you're not well prepared for the test. This may lead to cramming the night before, which will cause you to be physically and mentally exhausted for the test. Poor time management also contributes to feelings of stress, fear, and hopelessness as you realize you are not well prepared but don't know what to do about it.

Other times, test anxiety is not related to your preparation for the test but comes from unresolved fear. This may be a past failure on a test, or poor performance on tests in general. It may come from comparing yourself to others who seem to be performing better or from the stress of living up to expectations. Anxiety may be driven by fears of the future—how failure on this test would affect your educational and career goals. These fears are often completely irrational, but they can still negatively impact your test performance.

Elements of Test Anxiety

As mentioned earlier, test anxiety is considered to be an emotional state, but it has physical and mental components as well. Sometimes you may not even realize that you are suffering from test anxiety until you notice the physical symptoms. These can include trembling hands, rapid heartbeat, sweating, nausea, and tense muscles. Extreme anxiety may lead to fainting or vomiting. Obviously, any of these symptoms can have a negative impact on testing. It is important to recognize them as soon as they begin to occur so that you can address the problem before it damages your performance.

The mental components of test anxiety include trouble focusing and inability to remember learned information. During a test, your mind is on high alert, which can help you recall information and stay focused for an extended period of time. However, anxiety interferes with your mind's natural processes, causing you to blank out, even on the questions you know well. The strain of testing during anxiety makes it difficult to stay focused, especially on a test that may take several hours. Extreme anxiety can take a huge mental toll, making it difficult not only to recall test information but even to understand the test questions or pull your thoughts together.

Effects of Test Anxiety

Test anxiety is like a disease—if left untreated, it will get progressively worse. Anxiety leads to poor performance, and this reinforces the feelings of fear and failure, which in turn lead to poor performances on subsequent tests. It can grow from a mild nervousness to a crippling condition. If allowed to progress, test anxiety can have a big impact on your schooling, and consequently on your future.

Test anxiety can spread to other parts of your life. Anxiety on tests can become anxiety in any stressful situation, and blanking on a test can turn into panicking in a job situation. But fortunately, you don't have to let anxiety rule your testing and determine your grades. There are a number of relatively simple steps you can take to move past anxiety and function normally on a test and in the rest of life.

Physical Steps for Beating Test Anxiety

While test anxiety is a serious problem, the good news is that it can be overcome. It doesn't have to control your ability to think and remember information. While it may take time, you can begin taking steps today to beat anxiety.

Just as your first hint that you may be struggling with anxiety comes from the physical symptoms, the first step to treating it is also physical. Rest is crucial for having a clear, strong mind. If you are tired, it is much easier to give in to anxiety. But if you establish good sleep habits, your body and mind will be ready to perform optimally, without the strain of exhaustion. Additionally, sleeping well helps you to retain information better, so you're more likely to recall the answers when you see the test questions.

Getting good sleep means more than going to bed on time. It's important to allow your brain time to relax. Take study breaks from time to time so it doesn't get overworked, and don't study right before bed. Take time to rest your mind before trying to rest your body, or you may find it difficult to fall asleep.

Along with sleep, other aspects of physical health are important in preparing for a test. Good nutrition is vital for good brain function. Sugary foods and drinks may give a burst of energy but this burst is followed by a crash, both physically and emotionally. Instead, fuel your body with protein and vitamin-rich foods.

Also, drink plenty of water. Dehydration can lead to headaches and exhaustion, especially if your brain is already under stress from the rigors of the test. Particularly if your test is a long one, drink water during the breaks. And if possible, take an energy-boosting snack to eat between sections.

Along with sleep and diet, a third important part of physical health is exercise. Maintaining a steady workout schedule is helpful, but even taking 5-minute study breaks to walk can help get your blood pumping faster and clear your head. Exercise also releases endorphins, which contribute to a positive feeling and can help combat test anxiety.

When you nurture your physical health, you are also contributing to your mental health. If your body is healthy, your mind is much more likely to be healthy as well. So take time to rest, nourish your body with healthy food and water, and get moving as much as possible. Taking these physical steps will make you stronger and more able to take the mental steps necessary to overcome test anxiety.

Mental Steps for Beating Test Anxiety

Working on the mental side of test anxiety can be more challenging, but as with the physical side, there are clear steps you can take to overcome it. As mentioned earlier, test anxiety often stems from lack of preparation, so the obvious solution is to prepare for the test. Effective studying may be the most important weapon you have for beating test anxiety, but you can and should employ several other mental tools to combat fear.

First, boost your confidence by reminding yourself of past success—tests or projects that you aced. If you're putting as much effort into preparing for this test as you did for those, there's no reason you should expect to fail here. Work hard to prepare; then trust your preparation.

Second, surround yourself with encouraging people. It can be helpful to find a study group, but be sure that the people you're around will encourage a positive attitude. If you spend time with others who are anxious or cynical, this will only contribute to your own anxiety. Look for others who are motivated to study hard from a desire to succeed, not from a fear of failure.

Third, reward yourself. A test is physically and mentally tiring, even without anxiety, and it can be helpful to have something to look forward to. Plan an activity following the test, regardless of the outcome, such as going to a movie or getting ice cream.

When you are taking the test, if you find yourself beginning to feel anxious, remind yourself that you know the material. Visualize successfully completing the test. Then take a few deep, relaxing breaths and return to it. Work through the questions carefully but with confidence, knowing that you are capable of succeeding.

Developing a healthy mental approach to test taking will also aid in other areas of life. Test anxiety affects more than just the actual test—it can be damaging to your mental health and even contribute to depression. It's important to beat test anxiety before it becomes a problem for more than testing.

Study Strategy

Being prepared for the test is necessary to combat anxiety, but what does being prepared look like? You may study for hours on end and still not feel prepared. What you need is a strategy for test prep. The next few pages outline our recommended steps to help you plan out and conquer the challenge of preparation.

Step 1: Scope Out the Test

Learn everything you can about the format (multiple choice, essay, etc.) and what will be on the test. Gather any study materials, course outlines, or sample exams that may be available. Not only will this help you to prepare, but knowing what to expect can help to alleviate test anxiety.

Step 2: Map Out the Material

Look through the textbook or study guide and make note of how many chapters or sections it has. Then divide these over the time you have. For example, if a book has 15 chapters and you have five days to study, you need to cover three chapters each day. Even better, if you have the time, leave an extra day at the end for overall review after you have gone through the material in depth.

If time is limited, you may need to prioritize the material. Look through it and make note of which sections you think you already have a good grasp on, and which need review. While you are studying, skim quickly through the familiar sections and take more time on the challenging parts. Write out your plan so you don't get lost as you go. Having a written plan also helps you feel more in control of the study, so anxiety is less likely to arise from feeling overwhelmed at the amount to cover.

Step 3: Gather Your Tools

Decide what study method works best for you. Do you prefer to highlight in the book as you study and then go back over the highlighted portions? Or do you type out notes of the important information? Or is it helpful to make flashcards that you can carry with you? Assemble the pens, index cards, highlighters, post-it notes, and any other materials you may need so you won't be distracted by getting up to find things while you study.

If you're having a hard time retaining the information or organizing your notes, experiment with different methods. For example, try color-coding by subject with colored pens, highlighters, or post-it notes. If you learn better by hearing, try recording yourself reading your notes so you can listen while in the car, working out, or simply sitting at your desk. Ask a friend to quiz you from your flashcards, or try teaching someone the material to solidify it in your mind.

Step 4: Create Your Environment

It's important to avoid distractions while you study. This includes both the obvious distractions like visitors and the subtle distractions like an uncomfortable chair (or a too-comfortable couch that makes you want to fall asleep). Set up the best study environment possible: good lighting and a comfortable work area. If background music helps you focus, you may want to turn it on, but otherwise keep the room quiet. If you are using a computer to take notes, be sure you don't have any other windows open, especially applications like social media, games, or anything else that could distract you. Silence your phone and turn off notifications. Be sure to keep water close by so you stay hydrated while you study (but avoid unhealthy drinks and snacks).

Also, take into account the best time of day to study. Are you freshest first thing in the morning? Try to set aside some time then to work through the material. Is your mind clearer in the afternoon or evening? Schedule your study session then. Another method is to study at the same time of day that you will take the test, so that your brain gets used to working on the material at that time and will be ready to focus at test time.

Step 5: Study!

Once you have done all the study preparation, it's time to settle into the actual studying. Sit down, take a few moments to settle your mind so you can focus, and begin to follow your study plan. Don't give in to distractions or let yourself procrastinate. This is your time to prepare so you'll be ready to fearlessly approach the test. Make the most of the time and stay focused.

Of course, you don't want to burn out. If you study too long you may find that you're not retaining the information very well. Take regular study breaks. For example, taking five minutes out of every hour to walk briskly, breathing deeply and swinging your arms, can help your mind stay fresh.

As you get to the end of each chapter or section, it's a good idea to do a quick review. Remind yourself of what you learned and work on any difficult parts. When you feel that you've mastered the material, move on to the next part. At the end of your study session, briefly skim through your notes again.

But while review is helpful, cramming last minute is NOT. If at all possible, work ahead so that you won't need to fit all your study into the last day. Cramming overloads your brain with more information than it can process and retain, and your tired mind may struggle to recall even previously learned information when it is overwhelmed with last-minute study. Also, the urgent nature of cramming and the stress placed on your brain contribute to anxiety. You'll be more likely to go to the test feeling unprepared and having trouble thinking clearly.

So don't cram, and don't stay up late before the test, even just to review your notes at a leisurely pace. Your brain needs rest more than it needs to go over the information again. In fact, plan to finish your studies by noon or early afternoon the day before the test. Give your brain the rest of the day to relax or focus on other things, and get a good night's sleep. Then you will be fresh for the test and better able to recall what you've studied.

Step 6: Take a Practice Test

Many courses offer sample tests, either online or in the study materials. This is an excellent resource to check whether you have mastered the material, as well as to prepare for the test format and environment.

Check the test format ahead of time: the number of questions, the type (multiple choice, free response, etc.), and the time limit. Then create a plan for working through them. For example, if you have 30 minutes to take a 60-question test, your limit is 30 seconds per question. Spend less time on the questions you know well so that you can take more time on the difficult ones.

If you have time to take several practice tests, take the first one open book, with no time limit. Work through the questions at your own pace and make sure you fully understand them. Gradually work up to taking a test under test conditions: sit at a desk with all study materials put away and set a timer. Pace yourself to make sure you finish the test with time to spare and go back to check your answers if you have time.

After each test, check your answers. On the questions you missed, be sure you understand why you missed them. Did you misread the question (tests can use tricky wording)? Did you forget the information? Or was it something you hadn't learned? Go back and study any shaky areas that the practice tests reveal.

Taking these tests not only helps with your grade, but also aids in combating test anxiety. If you're already used to the test conditions, you're less likely to worry about it, and working through tests until you're scoring well gives you a confidence boost. Go through the practice tests until you feel comfortable, and then you can go into the test knowing that you're ready for it.

Test Tips

On test day, you should be confident, knowing that you've prepared well and are ready to answer the questions. But aside from preparation, there are several test day strategies you can employ to maximize your performance.

First, as stated before, get a good night's sleep the night before the test (and for several nights before that, if possible). Go into the test with a fresh, alert mind rather than staying up late to study.

Try not to change too much about your normal routine on the day of the test. It's important to eat a nutritious breakfast, but if you normally don't eat breakfast at all, consider eating just a protein bar. If you're a coffee drinker, go ahead and have your normal coffee. Just make sure you time it so that the caffeine doesn't wear off right in the middle of your test. Avoid sugary beverages, and drink enough water to stay hydrated but not so much that you need a restroom break 10 minutes into the test. If your test isn't first thing in the morning, consider going for a walk or doing a light workout before the test to get your blood flowing.

Allow yourself enough time to get ready, and leave for the test with plenty of time to spare so you won't have the anxiety of scrambling to arrive in time. Another reason to be early is to select a good seat. It's helpful to sit away from doors and windows, which can be distracting. Find a good seat, get out your supplies, and settle your mind before the test begins.

When the test begins, start by going over the instructions carefully, even if you already know what to expect. Make sure you avoid any careless mistakes by following the directions.

Then begin working through the questions, pacing yourself as you've practiced. If you're not sure on an answer, don't spend too much time on it, and don't let it shake your confidence. Either skip it and come back later, or eliminate as many wrong answers as possible and guess among the remaining ones. Don't dwell on these questions as you continue—put them out of your mind and focus on what lies ahead.

Be sure to read all of the answer choices, even if you're sure the first one is the right answer. Sometimes you'll find a better one if you keep reading. But don't second-guess yourself if you do immediately know the answer. Your gut instinct is usually right. Don't let test anxiety rob you of the information you know.

If you have time at the end of the test (and if the test format allows), go back and review your answers. Be cautious about changing any, since your first instinct tends to be correct, but make sure you didn't misread any of the questions or accidentally mark the wrong answer choice. Look over any you skipped and make an educated guess.

At the end, leave the test feeling confident. You've done your best, so don't waste time worrying about your performance or wishing you could change anything. Instead, celebrate the successful completion of this test. And finally, use this test to learn how to deal with anxiety even better next time.

Review Video: Test Anxiety
Visit mometrix.com/academy and enter code: 100340

Important Qualification

Not all anxiety is created equal. If your test anxiety is causing major issues in your life beyond the classroom or testing center, or if you are experiencing troubling physical symptoms related to your anxiety, it may be a sign of a serious physiological or psychological condition. If this sounds like your situation, we strongly encourage you to seek professional help.

Online Resources

Due to our efforts to try to keep this book to a manageable length, we've created a link that will give you access to all of your online resources:

mometrix.com/resources719/renalnutrition

It's Your Moment, Let's Celebrate It!

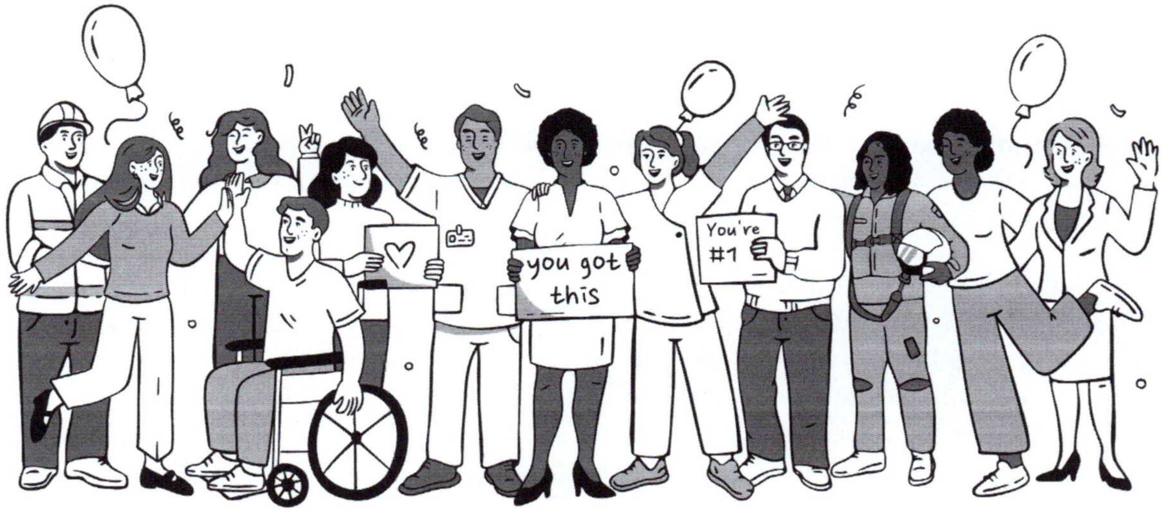

Share your story @mometrixtestpreparation